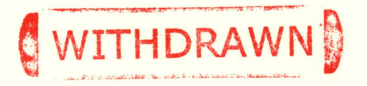

DRUGS AND SEX

DRUGS AND SEX

A BIBLIOGRAPHY

Compiled, with an introduction, by
Ernest L. Abel

GREENWOOD PRESS
WESTPORT, CONNECTICUT • LONDON, ENGLAND

Library of Congress Cataloging in Publication Data
Main entry under title:

Drugs and sex.

  Includes index.
  1. Generative organs—Effect of drugs on—Bibliography.
2. Psychotropic drugs—Physiological effect—
Bibliography.   3. Drugs and sex—Bibliography. I. Abel,
Ernest L., 1943-   . [DNLM: 1. Sex—Bibliography.
2. Sex behavior—Drug effects—Bibliography.   3. Psycho-
tropic drugs—Pharmacodynamics—Bibliography.   ZQV 77
A139d]
Z6663.R4D78   1983 [RM380]   016.615'78   83-5656
ISBN 0-313-23941-X (lib. bdg.)

Library of Congress Catalog Card Number: 83-5656
ISBN: 0-313-23941-X

First published in 1983

Greenwood Press
A division of Congressional Information Service, Inc.
88 Post Road West, Westport, Connecticut 06881

Printed in the United States of America

10 9 8 7 6 5 4 3 2 1

Contents

Introduction

The search for substances to enhance sexual drive has been relentless throughout recorded history. Ancient herbals, for example contain countless recipes for alleged aphrodisiacs. Very often, sexual power was attributed to these substances because they looked like sexual organs (for example, mandrake root), the idea being that "like affects like." Today, the consensus of opinion is that there is no such thing as an aphrodisiac. This opinion, however, is based on a concern with libido or performance. If subjective feelings such as enjoyment or pleasure are included in the criteria used to define aphrodisia, then this conclusion may have to be reassessed.

The list of substances that could possibly affect sexuality in all its ramifications is considerable. To deal with this vast body of information, some decision had to be made as to what to include and what to omit. A decision was arbitrarily made to include only psychoactive substances, that is, agents whose sites of action are primarily in the brain. This meant that hormones and antihormones and antihypertensive agents would not be included in the bibliography. A second decision excluded references to putative neurotransmitters and their precursors such as dopamine and l-dopa, since this would also take the listing too far afield. A third decision was made to omit articles appearing in the popular press, since inclusion of such articles would be haphazard and would also make the present task unmanageable.

The general format has been to list certain drugs and classes of drugs alphabetically, and within each class, to list pertinent references alphabetically by author. The index serves as a guide to specific items of interest within each drug category.

From an objective standpoint, very few studies have examined the effects of various agents on libido or sexual performance in any manner which resembles a scientific investigation. Most reports are anecdotal and come from clinical reports or "street lore." Studies in animals are suggestive, but such studies can only address the performance side of the issue or the physiological aspects of drug exposure (for example, hormonal levels, sperm motility). Prior to examining some of the literature in this area, the following considerations should be kept in mind in evaluating this subject area:

1) <u>Definitions</u>. Terms should be properly defined. "Impotence," for example, is frequently cited as being affected by various agents.

This term has been used as a synonym for decreased libido (sexual drive or interest), erectile dysfunction, or failure to ejaculate. The same is true of the term "frigidity" in terms of female sexuality and its counterparts.

2)"Set" and "setting." The conditions under which substances are taken will greatly affect their behavioral effects, especially at very low doses. "Set" refers to an individual's expectations. "Setting" refers to the environment in which a substance is taken. The effects of drugs such as marihuana, for example, are very much influenced by "set" and "setting."

3) Drug Dosage. The higher the drug dosage, the more likely its pharmacological actions will predominate over effects such as "set" and "setting."

4) Duration. The length of time a drug has been used is important since some drugs may not have been used long enough for their effects to manifest themselves.

5) Preexisting conditions. Prior sexual dysfunction is an important variable since such dysfunction may be attributed to a drug even though the condition was in existence before drug use began. Medical conditions such as hypertension are also associated with sexual dysfunction and must be taken into account when evaluating drug effects.

6) Age. The age of the user can be a factor since aging may be associated with decreased sexual activity and altered physiological response.

7) Multidrug use. The actions of one substance may be masked or enhanced by other substances. The user's history of drug usage is therefore important in evaluating the effect of a particular substance on sexual behavior or physiology.

8) General malaise. Sexual behavior may be affected by general listlessness associated with drug usage. This is an especially important consideration in evaluating studies in animals. In such studies an animal may appear to have lost interest in sex, but its real problem may be drug-induced malaise.

9) Methodology. Experimental studies should be conducted in which the investigators do not know what substances the subjects have received and the subjects do not know if they have received an active substance or a placebo. Subjects should also be randomly assigned to conditions and matched as closely as possible on all relevant variables. Such experimental conditions can rarely be met in a treatment situation, however. If they can be met, more confidence can be placed in the results.

MECHANISMS OF ACTION

There are a number of ways a drug may affect sexual function and physiology. General malaise, as already pointed out, can result in a decrease in all activity, including that associated with sex.

Studies in paraplegic animals and men, indicate that one way in which drugs may affect tumescence and ejaculation is through direct actions on spinal reflex centers underlying erectile and ejaculatory processes. Subarachnoid injection of alcohol, for example, has been used to inhibit priapism in paraplegic men.

The fact that a drug may inhibit penile tumescence or ejaculatory ability, however, does not necessarily mean that these vasomotor responses may not also be inhibited or stimulated secondarily through the actions of some agent on higher cortical centers or through hormonal mechanisms that underlie sexuality.

In many cases, drug use has been found to be associated with decreased levels of testosterone in men. Such decreases may be due to Leydig cell damage. However, Leydig cell damage does not preclude inhibition of the hypothamic-pituitary-gonadal axis as also being adversely affected as reflected in levels of luteinizing hormone.

Many substances may also produce impairment of spermatogenesis. Seminiferous tubules and tubular germinal layers may be adversely affected by drugs, and this could be reflected in impairment of spermatogenesis since spermatogonia arise from the tubular epithelium. Sterility may also result from direct actions on gonadal tissue or from obstruction of pathways through which sperm pass. Another possibility is that sperm motility may be affected due to direct actions on sperm or to effects on mucous secretion by the prostate or other organs such as the vas deferens.

Although much less work has been done on the effects of various agents on female sexuality and physiology, some work has begun to be done with respect to women and sex. In some cases, however, there is a definitional problem associated with terms such as promiscuity. Sexual promiscuity cannot be defined objectively, and as several authors have pointed out, however it is defined, it may be more characteristic of a particular subgroup of drug users than drug users as a whole.

Chronic use of certain drugs has been related to various obstetric and gynecological disorders such as menstrual problems and infertility. In many cases, however, it is not known whether these problems precipitated drug use or were precipitated by it. Studies in animals, however, have shown that in many cases, atrophy of ovaries, uterus, and fallopian tubes can occur following exposure to a variety of drugs. Various levels of hormones are also lowered in connection with the use of drugs. Such changes could result in decreased sexual responsiveness and impaired sexual physiology.

These considerations reflect certain generalities with respect to the actions of various agents on male and female sexuality. The following comments are directed at a more specific examination of the nature and the effects of the various substances cataloged in this bibliography.

ALCOHOL

Alcohol is a general term used to describe a class of compounds with a similar structure. It most cases, however, the compound being referred to is a specific member of this class, ethanol, which is also known as ethyl alcohol or grain alcohol.

Alcohol comes in the form of three main beverages--beer, wine, and distilled spirits. Beer contains about 3 to 6 percent alcohol; wine contains about 10 to 20 percent; and distilled spirits contain about 40 to 50 percent.

Alcohol is transported to all parts of the body, and it affects the functions of all parts of the body. However, its actions on the brain are the most apparent. Contrary to popular belief, alcohol is not a stimulant but a depressant. The apparent stimulant effect is due to early depression of inhibitory areas so that when these inhibitory areas are depressed, an apparent stimulation occurs.

In small amounts, alcohol is a euphoriant. Large amounts cause more and more depression, confusion, disorganization, loss of memory and perception, loss of coordination, and eventually loss of consciousness and death.

Despite its effects as a depressant, alcohol has been considered as an aphrodisiac for centuries. Possibly the most frequently quoted statement on its effects relating to sex is in Shakespeare's Macbeth (Act 2, scene 2): "It (alcohol) provokes and unprovokes: it provokes the desire, but it takes away from the performance."

Although there is no shortage of anecdotal information concerning alcohol's relation to sex, there is by contrast very little in the way of carefully controlled studies of this relation. Moreover, most of the available information concerns men. Very little has been done to investigate how alcohol affects female sexuality.

One of the more consistent findings with respect to alcohol and sexual function in men is that chronic alcoholism often results in impotence. In one study involving over 17,000 male alcoholics, about 8 percent were found to be impotent. Even after years of sobriety, about one-half of this number remained impotent, even though they still expressed a strong desire for sex. Another study reported a 31 percent incidence of erectile impotence and an 18 percent incidence of ejaculatory failure among a group of forty-five male alcoholics.

Controlled laboratory studies have corroborated these findings. Using college students and a penile strain gauge to measure tumescence, researchers have observed a dose-related inhibition in penile tumescence associated with ingestion of alcohol.

Studies on paraplegic animals and men suggest that one of the ways alcohol causes impotence is by affecting the spinal reflex centers underlying erectile and ejaculatory processes. In one study, for example, erectile and ejaculatory reflexes in dogs with midthoracic spinal transections were abolished by alcohol.

Although studies such as these indicate that alcohol can directly inhibit spinal neural mechanisms underlying tumescence and ejaculation, this does not preclude alcohol's affecting similar functions mediated by higher cortical centers or through hormonal mechanisms.

The relationship between alcohol consumption and hormonal mechanisms relating to sexual physiology has been actively studied in contrast to alcohol's effects on sexual behavior. In general, these studies have shown that chronic alcohol consumption often leads to feminization in men--for example, hypogonadism, gynecomastia, and decreased beard and pubic hair. Although such feminization may be the result of alcohol-related liver dysfunction, recent studies have shown that such changes can also occur independently of alcohol's effects on the liver.

A frequent observation among alcoholics and in animals chronically treated with alcohol is a decrease in serum testosterone levels. Clinical and experimental studies suggest that this decrease arises through a dual action of alcohol. On the one hand, alcohol appears to cause damage to the Leydig cells in the testes which are involved in the production of testosterone, and on the other, it appears to inhibit the hypothalamic-pituitary-gonadal axis by which the pituitary influences the testes to produce testosterone.

In terms of reproduction per se, one of the most important effects of chronic ingestion of alcohol is sperm damage. Alcohol not only inhibits sperm motility but also causes changes in sperm itself such

as curled tails, distended midsections, and broken heads. Sterility
may also occur as a direct result of alcohol's actions on gonadal
tissues or by causing obstruction of the vas deferens.

With respect to female sexuality, self-report studies of sexual
attitudes and behavior suggest that female alcoholics are more likely
to desire and engage in intercourse than nonalcoholics. A laboratory
study using the vaginal photoplethysmograph, an instrument to measure
vaginal pressure, indicated that alcohol causes a dose-related decrease
in vaginal pressure, but at the same time the women in this study stated
that they felt more sexually aroused with increasing blood alcohol
levels.

Chronic alcohol ingestion in women, as in men, results in various
adverse effects on reproductive physiology. Among the obstetrical
and gynecological problems related to alcohol consumption are menstrual disorders, miscarriage, infertility, and difficulties in labor.
Studies of animals have shown that chronic ingestion of alcohol can
result in atrophy of the ovary, uterus, and fallopian tubes.

AMPHETAMINES

Amphetamine is a general term for a class of drugs that causes
stimulation of the brain. These drugs are also called sympathomimetic
amines since they are similar in structure and function to endogenous
neuroamines. The three types of amphetamines are amphetamine sulfate (Benzedrine), dextroamphetmaine sulfate (Dexedrine), and methamphetamine hydrochloride (Methedrine). Methamphetamine is the most
potent and amphetamine sulfate the least potent of the series.

Amphetamines are used as mood elevators, energizers, antidepressants, appetite depressants, and as substances to promote
alertness. Among the slang terms used in connection with these substances are bennies, dexies, pep pills, hearts, meth, speed, splash,
and uppers.

The effects of amphetamines are believed to be due to their ability
to concentrate biogenic amines in the synapses by blocking their re-
uptake and enhancing their release. The general effect resulting from
this action is arousal. In the peripheral nervous system, amphetamines
cause constriction of blood vessels, increased heart rate, increased
blood pressure, and increased muscle tension. Extended use of amphetamines is associated with a number of adverse reactions including
insomnia, excessive talkativeness and motor activity, apprehension,
agitation, nervousness, and psychosis.

The reported effects of these drugs on sex have not been consistent.
In one study, increases, decreases, and no changes in libido were all
noted. Impotence and delayed ejaculation have also been reported in
men. Inconsistencies in effects have also been noted among women.
Some women have reported increased sexual feelings whereas others have
not. This variability may be due to a combination of dosage and
factors such as set and setting. As noted above, with low doses, subjective expectations and environmental factors exert themselves. Thus,
when men and women took relatively low doses, sexual feelings for both
were increased in one study, whereas with higher doses, impotence and
failure of orgasm were noted.

ANTIDEPRESSANTS

Antidepressants are mood elevators. They are generally divided into two main types, the tricyclic antidepressants such as amitriptyline hydrochloride (Elavil), and imipramine (Tofranil), and the monoamine oxidase inhibitors such as tranylcypromine (Parnate). These compounds are used for nonmedical purposes only to a minor extent since they have little impact on normal mood and they do not produce immediate pleasureable sensations.

In some cases, use of these drugs has been associated with decreased libido, decreased erection, and inhibition of ejaculation. Few reports concerning effects in women have been published, but in one study, women using monoamine oxidase inhibitors complained of difficulty in obtaining orgasm.

BARBITURATES

Barbiturates are sedative/hypnotic drugs. In small doses they sedate and relieve tension and anxiety. In larger doses, they induce sleep. Barbiturates are often divided into three classes according to their speed of elimination from the body. The ultrashort-acting barbiturates include sodium thiopental (Pentothal). These usually are eliminated by about three hours after intake. The short-to-intermediate barbiturates include secobarbital (Seconal), pentobarbital (Nembutal), and amobarbital (Amytal). These usually last for three to six hours. These are the most widely abused of the barbiturates. The third class are the long-lasting barbiturates including phenobarbital (Luminal) and barbital (Veronal). Their effects last from six to twenty-four hours. Slang terms for barbiturates include downers, goofballs, and a variety of color-related terms based on the color of the capsules they come in, for example, reds, yellows, blues, rainbows.

Barbiturates are among the most widely abused drugs. Patterns of use vary from chronic daily use of large doses to weekend binges. Consequences of high doses resemble that of alcohol and include initial euphoria, followed by impairment of memory and attention span, mental confusion, and motor incoordination. Acute barbiturate poisoning is one of the leading causes of drug-induced poisoning. Symptoms of barbiturate toxicity include excitement prior to sleep, coma, and respiratory failure.

There are relatively few reports of the effects of barbiturates on sexual behavior. In one study, male users reported an initial increase in libido followed by impotence and a decreased ability to maintain erection. In another study, a considerable number of barbiturate-dependent women claimed to be frigid and stopped having sexual relations with their husbands.

Very little information is available concerning how barbiturates affect sex hormones in humans. In female animals, barbiturates inhibit the surge of luteinizing hormone prior to ovulation, and as a result ovulation is blocked. In males, barbiturates produce decreases in levels of luteinizing hormone and decreases in testosterone levels.

BENZODIAZEPINES

Benzodiazepines are antianxiety drugs. The best known of these are Valium and Librium. The two other main drugs in this class are oxazepam (Serax) and chlorazepate (Tranxene).

Valium is now the most frequently prescribed drug in the United States. Although primarily used as an antianxiety drug, it is also a muscle relaxant and an anticonvulsant. The most common side effects of these drugs are drowsiness and weakness.

Surprisingly, there are very few reports of these drugs in connection with sex. In one study, a male using Librium had difficulty ejaculating. In another report, an individual complained of impotence. Considering the millions of people who use these drugs, the fact that there have been so few reports of sexual dysfunction in users suggests that they are relatively free of such actions.

CAFFEINE

Caffeine is a central nervous system stimulant. Caffeine is found in coffee, tea, chocolate, and in soft drinks. An average cup of coffee has about 100 mg of caffeine. Excessive use of caffeine is associated with dizziness, reflex hyperexcitability, heart palpitations, breathlessness, lightheadedness, nervousness, and irritability.

Although not generally considered to have sexual effects, there are reports of sexual arousal following ingestion of caffeine. This reaction, however, may be a general side effect of the overall stimulation produced by caffeine.

Studies in animals indicate that caffeine has a stimulatory effect on male sexual behavior in rats. Animals injected with caffeine approached females sooner and copulated with them sooner than did controls.

In humans, caffeine increases sperm motility and increases the longevity of sperm. A similar effect occurs in sperm from animals.

COCAINE

Cocaine is an alkaloid isolated from the coca plant. Pharmacologically, it is similar to the amphetamimes. Effects include euphoria, a sense of well-being, restlessness, and excitement. It is considered a central nervous system stimulant. Slang names for the drug include coke, snow, girl, dust, and big C. Chronic heavy use can result in nervousness, depression, and paranoia.

Cocaine rapidly enters the blood stream from all mucous membranes, including those in the nose. It is a potent constrictor of small blood vessels which accounts for the ulceration of the nasal lining in association with "snorting." Its stimulant action is in large part due to its inhibitory actions on the re-uptake of norepinephrine--a neurotransmitter--back into nerve endings after it has been released.

Cocaine has had a long historical association with sex. During the turn of the century it became popularly associated with excessive sexuality in many articles and books. Cocaine is still regarded as an aphrodisiac by many of its users. It is considered to intensify the sexual experience and increase sexual energy. In some cases it has been applied topically as a local anesthetic to prolong sex. Some studies support the belief that cocaine can increase sexual pleasure. In one study, for instance, male users reported prolonged sexual intercourse after cocaine use. Other studies report delayed orgasm and increased libido. Long-term studies of cocaine users report sexual stimulation in the absence of noteworthy sexual dysfunction.

LSD

LSD (lysergic acid diethylamine-25) is a white, odorless powder which has hallucinogenic effects. It produces alterations in consciousness and perceptions, although effects are highly variable. Unpleasant reactions include panic, anxiety, and confusion. Vivid images and thoughts are often experienced which may or may not be pleasureable.

Although praised as an aphrodisiac by some writers such as Timothy Leary, the reported effects of this drug on sex are inconsistent.

MARIHUANA

Marihuana refers to various preparations from the plant Cannabis sativa. Like alcohol, it is one of the oldest drugs known to man. The principal psychoactive ingredient in marihuana is delta-9-tetrahydro-cannabinol, a thick, viscous liquid which is insoluble in water.

The effects of marihuana are highly variable depending on dosage, previous experience of the user, set, setting, and various other factors. For most people, the main effects are euphoria, relaxation, altered perceptions, distortions of time and space, and loss of immediate memory. Adverse effects include acute panic reaction, incoordination, and bronchial congestion. There have been no deaths associated with marihuana use. Reported effects on chromosomes, brain damage, and immunity systems are inconsistent.

Marihuana has a long association with sex, but much of the available information concerning this association is anecdotal and contradictory. Marihuana is undeniably associated with increased sexual activity for many people, but this association is more likely due to a particular life style than to any pharmacological effects of the drug. The relation of marihuana to sex is very much related to dosage. At low doses, factors such as set and setting predominate, whereas at higher doses, the pharmacological actions of the drug become more important. Some attempts have been made to account for the reported enhancement of sexual enjoyment in terms of marihuana-induced changes in perception. By slowing down time perception, the impression of prolonged sexual involvement and orgasm may be created.

Studies in animals have not shed much light on the possible effects of marihuana on sex because marihuana is a general depressant in animals and all consummatory behavior is inhibited. The fact that most studies in animals report decreased sexual behavior may thus be due to a general malaise rather than any specific effect on such behavior.

Although initial studies suggested that marihuana lowered testosterone levels in men, these studies have not been corroborated and the weight of the evidence now suggests that marihuana does not significantly alter testosterone levels in men. In animals, however, decreases in testosterone levels following administration of marihuana have been consistently found.

Abnormal sperm production in marihuana users has been noted in several studies. In one study, about one-third the marihuana users had markedly reduced sperm counts. Among the reported aberrations in sperm observed in marihuana users are reduced nuclear size and disorganization of structure. Studies in animals have consistently shown testicular degenerations following marihuana exposure. In one study, daily administration of marihuana for thirty days caused seminiferous tubule degeneration and degeneration of sperm in dogs. In mice, daily administration of delta-9-tetrahydrocannabinol caused an increase in abnormal sperm, for example, heads lacking hooks, banana-shaped heads, and folded heads.

In one study, a number of marihuana users were reported to have developed gynecomastia (breasts). This report suggested the possibility that marihuana had feminizing-like effects. This report, however, has not been corroborated, and much of the evidence indicates that marihuana does not possess estrogenic activity.

Very little information is available concerning marihuana's effects in women. At the turn of the century, marihuana was frequently recommended for menstrual disorders, but there have been no current studies of marihuana in conjunction with menstruation except for a brief report which noted that marihuana users had shorter menstrual cycles than nonusers and had more menstrual cycles that were anovulatory or characterized by a shorter luteal phase.

Studies in animals have noted an adverse effect of marihuana on ovulation, and a decrease in luteinizing hormone levels.

METHAQUALONE

Methaqualone (Quallude, Sopor) is a sedative/hypnotic. It is similar to the barbiturates in effects. It was introduced into the United States in 1965 and at one time was the sixth most popular sedative/hypnotic in this country. Slang names for this drug include ludes, sopors, quads, and mandrakes.

Methaqualone has enjoyed a widespread use among high school and college students because of its alleged aphrodisiac properties. Among its other slang names, it was known as the "love drug," and "heroin for lovers." In one survey of college students, most women said they preferred it to marihuana. Among the reasons given for this preference were that it was said to increase sexual arousal, break down inhibitions, and cause relaxation. Men on the other hand, expressed a preference for marihuana over methaqualone, giving impotence as one of the reasons for this preference. Other studies, however, have reported opposite effects.

NARCOTICS

Narcotics such as morphine are derived from the opium poppy. Heroin is a derivative of morphine. Other narcotics such as methadone are synthetic opiates. Methadone has a potency somewhat similar to morphine but with a longer duration of action.

Like alcohol and marihuana, opium was one of the earliest psychoactive agents used by man. Descriptions of the behavioral effects of opium, for example, have been traced as far back as 4,000 B.C.

Opium is obtained from the poppy, Papaver somniferum, which

contains more than twenty alkaloids. The principal two alkaloids are morphine (about 10 percent) and codeine (0.5 percent). Morphine was isolated from opium in 1806. Heroin (diacetylmorphine) was produced in 1898 as a semisynthetic derivative of morphine.

Narcotic drugs have a variety of effects including analgesia, sedation, euphoria or dysphoria, respiratory depression, cough suppression, and antidiarrhea actions. The primary medical usage is relief from severe pain. Abuse is due to the euphoric sensation it produces, but this euphoria is not experienced by all users. Overdose can result in coma and death due to respiratory depression. Tolerance and dependence develop rapidly to these agents. Methadone is used extensively in treatment of withdrawal from heroin. Methadone prevents withdrawal, blocks the euphoria associated with heroin use, and reduces the craving for heroin. Methadone itself, however, can produce dependence. Other synthetic narcotics include pentazocine (Talwin) and meperidine (Demerol).

Early psychoanalytic thought equated injection of narcotics with sexual orgasm. Use of narcotics was therefore regarded as a means of sexual tension reduction. This was sometimes referred to in the clinical literature as a "pharmacogenic orgasm" and by users as a "rush."

Studies of heroin and methadone users, however, indicate that use of narcotics is related to decreased interest in sex, impotence, and delayed ejaculation. Interestingly, after recovery from addiction, respondents claim that their interest in sex is greater, and their sexual performance improved, over what it was prior to addiction.

Studies of secondary sex organs indicate that narcotics usage can result in impairment including decreased ejaculate volume and decreased seminal vesicular and prostatic secretions. Sperm count, for example, is often increased in narcotics users due to inadequate sperm dilution by these secondary sex organ secretions. Sperm motility is often decreased. In one study, ejaculate time was increased beyond twenty-five minutes, and in some cases it did not occur at all.

A large number of gynecological complaints are also associated with use of narcotics. Menstrual anomalies are very common among women narcotics users. In one study of female heroin users, 63 percent had amenorrhea. Menstrual anomalies tend to begin about two to twelve months after onset of use. By three months after abstinence, 43 percent of the women surveyed still continued to have menstrual dysfunction in one study. However, by about twelve months after abstinence, normal menstrual function returned for most women.

Studies of hormone levels in narcotics users have not always been consistent. In some cases, no changes in testosterone levels have been noted in heroin users. However, in most reports, a significant decrease in testosterone levels has been associated with opiate use.

NITRITES

Volatine nitrites such as amyl nitrite and isobutyl nitrite have frequently been mentioned in conjunction with sexual side effects. These are volatile liquids which are rapidly absorbed into the body by inhalation. They have been widely used to alter sensory perception, although originally they were introduced to relive chest pain.

Amyl nitrite (Vaporole, Aspirole) was sold in glass pearls which could be crushed in the hand, thereby allowing the liquid to be inhaled.

The drug causes dilation of coronary arteries, and this results in
greater perfusion and oxygenation of the heart. Smooth muscles in
other areas of the body are also relaxed.

Amyl nitrite causes time sense to slow down and results in a
feeling of fullness in the head. Sensory perceptions are said to be
increased in intensity.

Amyl nitrite has been especially used in connection with sex.
Very often the pearls are crushed just prior to climax to extend orgasm.
It is said to be used in this way especially among male homosexuals.
In one double-blind study, amyl nitrite was found to increase "sexual
passion" and decrease erection. Other reported effects include intensity of orgasm, prolonged orgasm, and delayed ejaculation. Among
the slang names used in connection with amyl nitrite are poppers,
pearls, snappers, and amys.

PHENCYCLIDINE

Phencyclidine was initially introduced as an analgesic but was
abandoned for accepted human usage following adverse reactions during
initial testing. The drug is inhaled, smoked when sprinkled on other
drugs such as marihuana, swallowed, or injected. It causes a variety
of effects including increased heart rate, increased deep reflexes,
sweating, flushing, dizziness, loss of coordination, and euphoria.
Slang names for this drug include PCP, angel dust, and hog.

Although not used primarily for sexual purposes, there are a
number of reports of sexual effects in users. In one study, light
users reported sexual dysfunction in connection with the drug, whereas
heavy users reported increased sexual excitement. Erectile and
ejaculatory failure have not been reported with low doses, but impairment has been noted in connection with high doses. While enhancement
of orgasm has not been noted, an alteration in the perception of
orgasm consisting of prolonged orgasm was noted by some users.

TOBACCO

Tobacco is a flowering perennial plant which is cultivated in
nearly every country of the world. The main component in tobacco
smoke that is believed responsible for its behavioral effects is
nicotine.

Nicotine is a colorless to pale yellow fluid which is very soluble
in water and lipids. It has a low boiling point and therefore
vaporizes readily as tobacco burns during the smoking process. As
a result of its solubility, it is rapidly distributed throughout all
tissues and fluids of the body, including the brain.

Nicotine is an excitor of a group of cholinergic neurotransmitter
receptors. Nicotine depolarizes these receptors, thereby initiating
nerve stimulation. This stimulation is followed by a blockade of
these same receptors resulting in a decrease in nerve activity. In
addition, nicotine stimulates the release of adrenaline from the adrenal
glands. This results in an increase in heart rate and vasoconstriction.

There is some clinical evidence that smoking may be associated
with impotence in some males. In one study, two men who consulted
a clinic because of erectile dysfunction, were advised to stop
smoking. Abstention for a few days resulted in restoration of penile

erectile function. Physiological tests suggested that the problem may have been the result of impairment of penile blood pressure increases due to smoking.

Several clinical studies also suggest that sperm motility may be adversely affected by smoking. In many studies, sperm motility has been found to be significantly lower among smokers. When these men abstained from smoking, sperm motility increased for many. Resumption of smoking once again resulted in a decrease in sperm motility.

Studies in animals of nicotine's effects on male sexual behavior and physiology have been inconclusive. Decreases in sexual activity or changes in reproductive organs, for example, have been attributed in many instances to the indirect effects of nicotine on food consumption or to drug-related general malaise.

There is virtually no information, anecdotal or otherwise, concerning tobacco's effects on female sexuality. Several studies in animals, however, have suggested that chronic exposure to cigarette smoking or nicotine can adversely affect ovarian function and can affect the release of hormones involved in ovulation in animals. Several studies have also documented an earlier onset of menopause in women who smoke. One study, for example, found that menopause occurred at 49.4 years of age for a group of nonsmokers, at 48.0 years for women who smoked one to fourteen cigarettes per day, and at 47.6 years for women who smoked fifteen or more cigarettes a day. One of the explanations for this finding was that smoking may directly affect ovarian function.

DRUGS AND SEX

Alcohol

1. ABEL, E.L. (1980) 'A review of alcohol's effects on sex and
         reproduction.' Drug and Alcohol Dependence, 5, 321-332.

2. AKHTAR, M.J. (1977) 'Sexual disorders in male alcoholics.'
         In: J.S. Madden, R. Walker, and W.H. Kenyon, eds. Alco-
         holism and Drug Dependence: A Multidisciplinary Approach.
         New York: Plenum Press, pp. 3-12.

3. AL-HUSSAINY, T.H., MOSA, S.O., and AL-JIBOORI, N.A. (1982)
         'Effect of ethyl alcohol on the female reproductive per-
         formance and fetal development of albino mice.' Feder-
         ation Proceedings, 41, 1465 (abstract).

4. AMELAR, R.D., DUBIN, L., and SCHOENFELD, C. (1980) 'Sperm
         motility.' Fertility and Sterility, 34, 197-215.

5. ANDERSON, R.A., JR., REDDY, J.M., OSWALD, C., WILLIS, B., and
         ZANEVELD, L.J.D. (1980) 'Decreased male fertility
         induced by chronic alcohol ingestion.' Federation Pro-
         ceedings; Federation of American Societies for Exper-
         imental Biology, 39 (abstract).

6. ANDERSON, R.A., JR., WILLIS, B.R., OSWALD, C., GUPTA, A., and
         ZANEVELD, L.J.D. (1981) 'Delayed male sexual maturation
         induced by chronic ethanol ingestion.' Federation Pro-
         ceedings; Federation of American Societies for Exper-
         imental Biology, 40, 825 (abstract).

7. ANDERSON, R.A., JR., WILLIS, B.R., OSWALD, C., REDDY, J.M., BEY-
         LER, S.A., and ZANEVELD, L.J.D. (1980) 'Hormonal im-
         balance and alterations in testicular morphology induced
         by chronic ingestion of ethanol.' Biochemical Pharmacol-
         ogy, 29, 1409-1419.

8. ANONYMOUS. (1949) 'Effect of alcohol and tobacco on fertility.'
         (Any Questions?) British Medical Journal, 2, 768.

9. ANONYMOUS. (1955) 'Chronic alcoholism and fertility.' (Any
         Questions?) British Medical Journal, 1, 1170.

10. ANONYMOUS. (1975) 'Libido of female alcoholics.' (Questions
     and Answers.) Medical Aspects of Human Sexuality, 9, 99.

11. ANONYMOUS. (1980) 'Alcohol and sex.' Bottom Line, 3, 17-18.

12. ARLITT, A.H., and WELLS, H.G. (1917) 'The effect of alcohol on
     the reproductive tissues.' Journal of Experimental Med-
     icine, 26, 769-782.

13. ARON, E., FLANZY, M., COMBESCOT, C., PUISAIS, J., DEMARET, J.,
     REYNOUARD-BRAULT, F., and IGERT, C. (1965) 'L'alcool est-
     il dans le vin l'élément qui perturbe, chez la ratte, le
     cycle vaginal?' ['Is alcohol the element in wine which
     disturbs the estrous cycle in the rat?'] Bulletin de
     l'Académie Nationale de Médecine, 149, 112-120.

14. ATHANASIOU, R., SHAVER, P., and TAVRIS, C. (1970) 'Sex: A
     Psychology Today report on more than 20,000 responses to
     101 questions on sexual attitudes and practices.' Psy-
     chology Today, 4, 39.

15. BADR, F.M., and BADR, R.S. (1975) 'Induction of dominant lethal
     mutation in male mice by ethyl alcohol.' Nature, 253, 134-
     136.

16. BADR, F.M., and BARTKE, A. (1974) 'Effect of ethyl alcohol on
     plasma testosterone level in mice.' Steroids, 23, 921-927.

17. BADR, F.M., BARTKE, A., DALTERIO, S., and BULGER, W. (1977)
     'Suppression of testosterone production by ethyl alcohol:
     Possible mode of action.' Steroids, 30, 647-655.

18. BADR, F.M., SMITH, M.S., DALTERIO, S.L., and BARTKE, A. (1979)
     'Role of the pituitary and the adrenals in mediating the
     effects of alcohol on testicular steroidogenesis in mice.'
     Steroids, 34, 477-482.

19. BAHNSEN, M., GLUUD, C., JOHNSEN, S.G., BENNETT, P., SVENSTRUP,
     S., MICIC, S., DIETRICHSON, O., SVENDSEN, L.B., and BRODT-
     HAGEN, U.A. (1981) 'Pituitary-testicular function in
     patients with alcoholic cirrhosis of the liver.' European
     Journal of Clinical Investigation, 11, 473-479.

20. BAKER, H., BERGER, H.G., DEKRETSER, D.M., DULMANIS, A., HARTSON,
     B., O'CONNOR, S., PAULSEN, C.A., PURECELL, N., RENNIE, G.C.,
     SCAH, C.S., TAFT, H.P., and WANG, C. (1976) 'A study of
     the endocrine manifestations of hepatic cirrhosis.' Quart-
     erly Journal of Medicine, 45, 145-178.

21. BALABAUD, C., MAGNE, F., SARIC, J., and BIOULAC, P. (1981)
     'Alcohol and hypogonadism.' Gastroenterology, 80, 882.

22. BARK, N. (1979) 'Fertility and ofspring of alcoholic women:
     An unsuccessful search for the fetal alcohol syndrome.'
     British Journal of Addiction, 74, 43-49.

23.   BECKMAN, L.J.   (1978)   'Sex-role conflict in alcoholic women:
      Myth or reality.'   Journal of Abnormal Psychology, 87, 408-
      417.

24.   BECKMAN, L.J.   (1979)   'Reported effects of alcohol on the sex-
      ual feelings and behavior of women alcoholics and nonalco-
      holics.'   Journal of Studies on Alcohol, 40, 272-282.

25.   BELFER, M.L., SHADER, R.I., CARROLL, M., and HARMATZ, J.S.
      (1971)   'Alcoholism in women.'   Archives of General Psy-
      chiatry, 25, 540-544.

26.   BENEDIK, T.G.   (1972)   'Food and drink as aphrodisiacs.'   Sexual
      Behavior, 2, 5-10.

27.   BERENSON, D.   (1976)   'Sexual counseling with alcoholics.'   In:
      J. Newman, ed.   Sexual Counseling for Persons with Alcohol
      Problems: Proceedings of a Workshop.   Pittsburgh, Penn-
      sylvania: Western Pennsylvania Institute of Alcohol Stud-
      ies, University of Pittsburgh.

28.   BERTHOLET, E.   (1909)   'Über Atrophie des Hodens bei chronischem
      Alkoholismus.'   ['Regarding the atrophy of the testicle in
      chronic alcoholism.']   Zentralblatt für Allgemeine Path-
      ologie und Pathologische Anatomie, 20, 1062-1066.

29.   BERTHOLET, E.   (1912)   'Alterations anatomo-pathologique, ob-
      servées à l'autopsie de 100 alcoolique chroniques.'   ['Ana-
      tomopathological alterations, observed in the autopsy of
      100 chronic alcoholics.']   Bericht über den XIII. Inter-
      nationalen Kongress gegen den Alkoholismus, 13, 181-186.

30.   BERTHOLET, F.   (1913)   Action de l'alcoolisme chronique sur les
      organes de l'homme et sur les glandes reporcutives en par-
      ticular.   [The Action of Chronic Alcoholism on the Organs
      of the Male and on the Reproductive Glands in Particular.]
      Lausanne.

31.   BHALLA, V.K., CHEN, C.J.H., and GNANAPRAKASAM, M.S.   (1979)
      'Effects of in vivo administration of human chorionic
      gonadotropin and ethanol on the processes of testicular
      receptor depletion and replenishment.'   Life Sciences,
      24, 1315-1323.

32.   BLAKE, C.A.   (1974)   'Centrally acting drugs must inhibit spon-
      taneous neural stimulation of luteinizing hormone release
      for a specific 7-hour period to block ovulation in rats.'
      Federation Proceedings; Federation of American Societies
      for Experimental Biology, 33 (Part 1), 221 (abstract).

33.   BLAKE, C.A.   (1974)   'Differentiation between the "critical per-
      iod," the "activation period" and the "potential activation
      period" for neurohumoral stimulation of LH release in pro-
      estrous rats.'   Endocrinology, 95, 572-578.

34. BLAKE, C.A. (1974) 'Localization of the inhibitory actions of
     ovulation-blocking drugs on release of luteinizing hormone
     in ovariectomized rats.' Endocrinology, 95, 999-1004.

35. BLAKE, C.A. (1978) 'Paradoxical effects of drugs acting on the
     central nervous system on the preovulatory release of pit-
     uitary luteinizing hormone in pro-oestrous rats.' Journal
     of Endocrinology, 79, 319-326.

36. BOGGAN, W.O., RANDALL, C.L., and DODDS, H.M. (1979) 'Delayed
     sexual maturation in female C57BL/6J mice prenatally ex-
     posed to alcohol.' Research Communications in Chemical
     Pathology and Pharmacology, 23, 117-125.

37. BOUIN, P., and GARNIER, C. (1900) 'Alterations du tube sémin-
     ifère au cours de l'alcoolisme expérimental chez le rat
     blanc.' ['Alterations in the seminiferous tubule in the
     course of experimental alcoholism in the white rat.']
     Comptes Rendus des Seances de la Société de Biologie et
     de Ses Filiales, 52, 23.

38. BOYDEN, T.W., SILVERT, M.A., and PAMENTER, R.W. (1981) 'Acet-
     aldehyde acutely impairs canine testicular testosterone
     secretion.' European Journal of Pharmacology, 70, 571-576.

39. BRIDDELL, D.W., RIMM, D.C., CADDY, G.R., KRAWITZ, G., SHOLIS, D.,
     and WUNDERLIN, R.J. (1978) 'Effects of alcohol and cogni-
     tive set on sexual arousal to deviant stimuli.' Journal of
     Abnormal Psychology, 87, 418-430.

40. BRIDDELL, D.W., and WILSON, G.T. (1976) 'Effects of alcohol
     and expectancy set on male sexual arousal.' Journal of
     Abnormal Psychology, 85, 225-234.

41. BRZEK, A. (1977) 'Male sexuality and alcohol.' Casopis Lekaru
     Ceskoslovenska, 116, 1024-1026.

42. BRZEK, A., SKALÁ, J., and LACHMAN, M. (1978) 'Spermabefunde
     bei Alkoholikern.' ['Spermatologic findings in alcoho-
     lics.'] Dermatologische Monatsschrift, 164, 557-559.

43. BRZEK, A., SKALÁ, J., and LACHMAN, M. (1980) 'Změny spermato-
     logických nálezů během protialkoholní léčby.' ['Spermato-
     logic parameter changes in the course of alcoholism treat-
     ment.'] Protialkoholicky Obzor, 15, 15-18.

44. BURTON, G., and KAPLAN, H.M. (1968) 'Sexual behavior and
     adjustment of married alcoholics.' Quarterly Journal of
     Studies on Alcoholism, 29, 603-609.

45. CENI, C. (1904) 'Influenza dell'alcoolismo sul potere di 'pro-
     creare e sui discendenti.' ['The influence of alcohol on
     the ability to reproduce and on the descendants.']
     Rivista Sperimentelle di Freniatria, 30, 339-353.

46. CERUL, M. (1976) 'Basic considerations in sexual counseling.'
     In: J. Newman, ed. Sexual Counseling for Persons with
     Alcohol Problems. Pittsburgh, Pennsylvania: University
     of Pittsburgh, pp. 24-47.

47. CHAPIN, R.E., BREESE, G.R., and MUELLER, R.A. (1980) 'Possible
     mechanisms of reduction of plasma luteinizing hormone by
     ethanol.' Journal of Pharmacology and Experimental Ther-
     apeutics, 212, 6-10.

48. CHAUDHURY, R.R., and MATTHEWS, M. (1966) 'Effect of alcohol
     on the fertility of female rabbits.' Journal of Endocrin-
     ology, 34, 275-276.

49. CHAUHAN, P.S., ARAVINDAKSHAN, M., KUMAR, N.S., and SUNDARAM, K.
     (1980) 'Failure of ethanol to induce dominant lethal
     mutations in Wistar male rats.' Mutation Research, 79,
     263-275.

50. CHEN, J.J., and SMITH, E.R. (1979) 'Effects of perinatal alco-
     hol on sexual differentiation and open-field behavior in
     rats.' Hormones and Behavior, 13, 219-231.

51. CICERO, T.J. (1980) 'Sex differences in the effects of alcohol
     and other psychoactive drugs on endocrine function: Clin-
     ical and experimental evidence.' In: O.J. Kalant, ed.
     Research Advances in Alcohol and Drug Problems. New York:
     Plenum Press, pp. 545-593.

52. CICERO, T.J. (1981) 'Pathogenesis of alcohol-induced endocrine
     abnormalities.' Advances in Alcohol and Substance Abuse,
     1, 87-112.

53. CICERO, T.J. (1982) 'Alcohol effects on the endocrine system.'
     In: Alcohol and Health. Monograph No. 2: Biomedical
     Processes and Consequences of Alcohol Use. U.S. Department
     of Health, Education, and Human Services. Rockville, Mary-
     land: National Institute on Alcohol Abuse and Alcoholism,
     pp. 53-94.

54. CICERO, T.J. (1982) 'Alcohol-induced deficits in the hypo-
     thalamic-pituitary-luteinizing hormone axis in the male.'
     Alcoholism: Clinical and Experimental Research, 6, 207-215.

55. CICERO, T.J., and BADGER, T.M. (1977) 'Effects of alcohol on
     the hypothalamic-pituitary-gonadal axis in the male rat.'
     Journal of Pharmacology and Experimental Therapeutics, 201,
     427-433.

56. CICERO, T.J., and BELL, R.D. (1979) 'Acetaldehyde directly in-
     hibits the conversion of androstenedione to testosterone in
     the testes.' Third International Symposium on Alcohol and
     Aldehyde Metabolizing Systems, p. 17 (abstract).

57. CICERO, T.J., and BELL, R.D.   (1980) 'Effects of ethanol and
       acetaldehyde on the biosynthesis of testosterone in the
       rodent testes.' Biochemical and Biophysical Research Com-
       munications, 94, 814-819.

58. CICERO, T.J., BELL, R.D., and BADGER, T.M.   (1980) 'Acetalde-
       hyde directly inhibits the conversion of androstenedione
       to testosterone in the testes.' In: Alcohol and Acetalde-
       hyde Metabolizing Systems-IV. Volume 132: Advances in
       Experimental Medicine and Biology. Ed. R.G. Thurman.
       New York: Plenum Press, 211-217.

59. CICERO, T.J., BELL, R.D., and BADGER, T.M.   (1980) 'Multiple
       effects of ethanol on the hypothalamic-pituitary gonadal
       axis in the male.' In: Biological Effects of Alcohol:
       Proceedings of the International Symposium on Biological
       Research in Alcoholism, Zurich, Switzerland (June, 1978).
       Ed. Henri Begleiter. New York: Plenum Press, pp. 463-
       478.

60. CICERO, T.J., BELL, R.D., and MEYER, E.R.   (1979) 'Direct ef-
       fects of ethanol and acetaldehyde on testicular steroido-
       genesis.' Federation Proceedings, 38, 428 (abstract).

61. CICERO, T.J., BELL, R.D., MEYER, E.R., and BADGER, T.M.   (1980)
       'Ethanol and acetaldehyde directly inhibit testicular
       steroidogenesis.' Journal of Pharmacology and Experimen-
       tal Therapeutics, 213, 228-233.

62. CICERO, T.J., BERNSTEIN, D., and BADGER, T.M.   (1978) 'Effects
       of acute alcohol administration on reproductive endocrin-
       ology in the male rat.' Alcoholism: Clinical and Exper-
       imental Research, 2, 249-254.

63. CICERO, T.J., MEYER, E.R., and BELL, R.D.   (1979) 'Effects of
       ethanol on the hypothalamic-pituitary-luteinizing hormone
       axis and testicular steroidogenesis.' Journal of Phar-
       macology and Experimental Therapeutics, 208, 210-215.

64. CICERO, T.J., NEWMAN, K.S., and MEYER, E.R.   (1981) 'Ethanol-
       induced inhibitions of testicular steroidogenesis in the
       male rat: Mechanisms of actions.' Life Science (Oxford),
       28, 871-877.

65. CLARK, R.A.   (1952) 'The projective measurement of experimental-
       ly induced levels of sexual motivation.' Journal of Exper-
       imental Psychology, 44, 391-399.

66. CLARK, R.A., and SENSIBAR, M.R.   (1955) 'The sexual relation-
       ship between symbolic and manifest projections of sexual-
       ity with some incidental correlates.' Journal of Abnormal
       and Social Psychology, 50, 327-334.

67. COBB, C.F., ENNIS, M.F., VAN THIEL, D.H., GAVALER, J.S., and LESTER, R. (1978) 'Acetaldehyde and ethanol are direct testicular toxins.' Surgical Forum, 29, 641-644.

68. COBB, C.F., ENNIS, M.F., VAN THIEL, D.H., GAVALER, J.S., and LESTER, R. (1979) 'Alcohol: Its effect on the isolated perfused rat testes.' Alcoholism: Clinical and Experimental Research, 3, 171 (abstract).

69. COBB, C.F., ENNIS, M.F., VAN THIEL, D.H., GAVALER, J.S., and LESTER, R. (1980) 'Isolated testes perfusion: A method using a cell- and protein-free perfusate useful for the evaluation of potential drug and/or metabolic injury.' Metabolism, 29, 71-79.

70. COBB, C.F., GAVALER, J.S., and VAN THIEL, D.H. (1981) 'Is ethanol a testicular toxin?' Clinical Toxicology, 18, 149-154.

71. COBB, C.F., VAN THIEL, D.H., ENNIS, M.F., GAVALER, J.S., and LESTER, B. (1978) 'Acetaldehyde and ethanol are testicular toxins.' Gastroenterology, 75, 958 (abstract).

72. CORDES, H. (1898) 'Untersuchungen über den Einfluss acuter und chronischer Allgemeinerkrankungen auf die Testikel, special auf die Spermatogenese, sowie Beobachtungen über das Auftreten von Fett in den Hoden.' ['Studies on the influence of acute and chronic general illnesses in the testicle, especially on spermatogenesis, as well as observations on the occurrence of fat in the testicle.'] Virchow's Archiv, 151, 402.

73. CROWLEY, T.J., STYNES, A.J., HYDINGER, M., and KAUFMAN, I.C. (1974) 'Ethanol, methamphetamine, pentobarbital, morphine, and monkey social behavior.' Archives of General Psychiatry, 31, 829-838.

74. CURLEE, J. (1969) 'Alcoholism and the "empty nest."' Bulletin of the Meninger Clinic, 33 165.

75. CURRAN, F.J. (1937) 'Personality studies in alcoholic women.' Journal of Nervous and Mental Disease, 86, 645.

76. CUST, G. (1981) 'Smoking, drinking, eating, and sex--Some practical aspects of preventing deaths from cancer.' Practitioner, 225, 853-856.

77. CUTLER, M.G. (1976) 'Changes in the social behavior of laboratory mice during administration and on withdrawal from non-ataxic doses of ethyl alcohol.' Neuropharmacology (Oxford), 15, 495-498.

78. DANFORTH, C.H. (1919) 'Evidence that germ cells are subject to selection on the bases of their genetic patient abilities.' Journal of Experimental Zoology, 28, 385-412.

79. DAVIS, R.   (1914) 'The effect of alcohol on the male germ cells, studied by means of double matings.' Science, New Series, 39, 476-477.

80. DEVITO, R.A., and MAROZAS, R.J.   (1981) 'The alcoholic satyr.' Sexuality and Disability, 4, 234-245.

81. DEWSBURY, D.A.   (1967) 'Effects of alcohol ingestion on copulatory behavior of male rats.' Psychopharmacologie (Berlin), 11, 276-281.

82. DISTILLER, L.A., SAGEL, J., DUBOWITZ, B., KAY, G., CARR, P.J., KATZ, M., and KEW, M.C.   (1976) 'Pituitary-gonadal function in men with alcoholic cirrhosis of the liver.' Hormone and Metabolism Research, 8, 461-465.

83. DIXIT, V.P., AGRAWAL, M., and LOHIYA, N.K.   (1976) 'Effects of a single ethanol injection into the vas deferens on the testicular function of rats.' Endokrinologie (Leipzig), 67, 8-13.

84. DOEPFMER, R., and HINCKERS, H.J.   (1965) 'Zur Frage der Keimschädigung im akuten Rausch.' ['On the question of germ-cell damage in acute alcohol intoxication.'] Zeitschrift für Haut und Geschlechtskrankheiten, 39, 94-107.

85. DOEPFMER, R., and HINCKERS, H.J.   (1966) 'Zur Frage der Alkoholeinwirkung auf die Motilität menschlicher Spermien.' ['On the question of alcohol action on the mobility of human sperm.'] Zeitschrift für Haut und Geschlechtskrankheiten, 40, 378-382.

86. DOWSLING, J.L.   (1978) 'Sex therapy for recovering alcoholics: An essential part of family therapy.' International Journal of the Addictions, 15, 6.

87. DRIFE, J.O.   (1982) 'Drugs and sperm.' British Medical Journal, 284, 844.

88. DUDEK, F.A., and TURNER, D.S.   (1982) 'Alcoholism and sexual functioning.' Journal of Psychoactive Drugs, 14, 47-54.

89. DUNGAY, N.S.   (1913) 'A study of the effects of injury upon the fertilizing power of sperm.' Biological Bulletin, 25, 213-216.

90. EAGON, P.K., PORTER, L.E., GAVALER, J.S., EGLER, K.M., and VAN THIEL, D.H.   (1981) 'Effect of ethanol feeding upon levels of a male-specific hepatic estrogen-binding protein: A possible mechanism for feminization.' Alcoholism: Clinical and Experimental Research, 5, 183-187.

91. ELLINGBOE, J., MENDELSON, J.H., KUEHNLE, J.C., SKUPNY, A.S.T., and MILLER, K.D. (1980) 'Effect of acute ethanol ingestion on integrated plasma prolactin levels in normal men.' Pharmacology, Biochemistry, and Behavior, 12, 297-301.

92. ELLINGBOE, J., and VARANELLI, C.C. (1979) 'Ethanol inhibits testosterone biosynthesis by direct action on Leydig cells.' Research Communications in Chemical Pathology and Pharmacology, 24, 87-102.

93. ENOS, W.F., and BEYER, J.C. (1980) 'Prostatic acid phosphatase, aspermia, and alcoholism in rape cases.' Journal of Forensic Science, 25, 353-356.

94. ESKAY, R.L., RYBACK, R.S., GOLDMAN, M., and MAJCHROWICZ, E. (1981) 'Effect of chronic ethanol administration on plasma levels of LH and the estrous cycle in the female rat.' Alcoholism: Clinical and Experimental Research, 5, 204-206.

95. EWING, J.A. (1968) 'Alcohol, sex, and marriage.' Medical Aspects of Human Sexuality, 4, 43-50.

96. FABRE, L.F., PASCO, P.J., LIEGEL, J.M., and FARMER, R.W. (1973) 'Abnormal testosterone excretion in men alcoholics.' Quarterly Journal of Studies on Alcoholism, 34, 57-63.

97. FAHIM, M.S., DEMENT, G., and HALL, D.G. (1970) 'Induced alterations in hepatic metabolism of androgens in the rat.' American Journal of Obstetrics and Gynecology, 107, 1085-1091.

98. FARKAS, G.M., and ROSEN, R.C. (1976) 'Effect of alcohol on elicited male sexual response.' Journal of Studies on Alcohol, 37, 265-272.

99. FARMER, R.W., and FABRE, L.F., JR. (1975) 'Some endocrine aspects of alcoholism.' Advances in Experimental Medical Biology, 56, 277-289.

100. FARNSWORTH, W.E., CAVANAUGH, A.H., BROWN, J.R., ALVAREZ, I., and LEWANDOWSKI, L.M. (1978) 'Factors underlying infertility in the alcoholic.' Archives of Andrology, 1, 193-195.

101. FARRELL, J.I. (1938) 'The secretion of alcohol by the genital tract: An experimental study.' Journal of Urology, 40, 62-65.

102. FARRY, K., and TITTMAR, H.-G. (1975) 'Alcohol as a teratogen: Effects of maternal administration in rats on sexual development in female offspring.' Pharmacology, Reproduction, Obstetrics and Gynecology, 3, 619-620.

103.   FICHER, M., and LEVITT, D.R.   (1980)   'Testicular dysfunction
        and sexual impotence in the alcoholic rat.'   Journal of
        Steroid Biochemistry, 13, 1089-1095.

104.   FIGUERIDO, C.A.   (1947)   'Los llamados males germinales y los
        descendientes de toxicomanos.'   ['So-called germ damage
        and the offspring of addicts.']   Revista de Sanidad
        Higiene Publica (Madrid), 21, 1215-1221.

105.   FISHER, M., and LEVITT, D.R.   (1978)   'Effects of alcohol on
        rat testicular steroidogenesis.'   Sixtieth Annual Meeting--
        Endocrinology Society, Miami, Florida.

106.   FLEIT, L.   (1979)   Alcohol and Sexuality: A Handbook for the
        Counselor/Therapist.   Arlington, Virginia: H/P Publishing
        Company.

107.   FRANEK, B., and FRANEK, M.   (1981)   'Sexual rehabilitation in
        alcoholism recovery.'   27th International Institute on
        the Prevention and Treatment of Alcoholism, Vienna, Aus-
        tria, June 15-20, 1981, pp. 273-285.

108.   FRANEK, B., and FRANEK, H.   (1982)   'Sexual rehabilitation in
        alcoholism recovery.'   Alcoholism: Clinical and Exper-
        imental Research, 6, 141 (abstract).

109.   FREEMAN, C.   (1975)   'Preliminary human trial of a new male
        sterilization procedure: Vas sclerosing.'   Fertility and
        Sterility, 26, 162-166.

110.   FREEMAN, C., and COFFEY, D.S.   (1973)   'Male sterility induced
        by ethanol injection into the vas deferens.'   Internation-
        al Journal of Fertility, 18, 129-132.

111.   FREEMAN, C. and COFFEY, D.S.   (1973)   'Sterility in male ani-
        mals induced by injection of chemical agents into the vas
        deferens.'   Fertility and Sterility, 24, 884-890.

112.   FRETS, G.P.   (1931)   Alcohol and the Other Germ Poisons.
        Nijhoff: The Hague.

113.   FUEYO-SILVA, A., MENÉNDEZ-PATTERSON, A., and MARIN, B.   (1980)
        'Efectos del consumo prenatal del alcohol sobre la fecun-
        didad, natalidad, crecimiento, apertura vaginal y ciclo
        sexual en la rata.'   ['Effects of prenatal alcohol consump-
        tion upon fecundity, natality, growth, vaginal opening,
        and sexual cycle in the rat.']   Reproduccion, 4, 265-270.

114.   FUKUDA, Y., and TOYODA, Y.   (1974)   'Effects of oral adminis-
        tration of ethanol on ovulation and embryonic development
        in the rat.'   Japanese Journal of Fertility and Sterility,
        19, 46-52.

115.   GALLANT, D.M.   (1968)   'The effect of alcohol and drug abuse on
       sexual behavior.'   Medical Aspects of Human Sexuality, 2,
       30-36.

116.   GALVÃO-TELES, A., ANDERSON, D.C., BURKE, C.W., and MARSHALL,
       J.C.   (1973)   'Biologically active androgens and oestra-
       diol in men with chronic liver disease.'   Lancet (London),
       1, 173-177.

117.   GANTT, W.H.   (1952)   'Effect of alcohol in the sexual reflexes
       of normal and neurotic male dogs.'   Psychosomatic Med-
       icine, 14, 174-181.

118.   GAVALER, J.S., VAN THIEL, D.H., and LESTER, R.   (1980)
       'Ethanol: A gonadal toxin in the mature rat of both
       sexes.'   Alcoholism: Clinical and Experimental Research,
       4, 271-276.

119.   GEE, W.   (1916)   'Effects of acute alcoholization on the germ
       cells of fundulus heteroclitus.'   Biological Bulletin, 31,
       297-406.

120.   GODLEWSKI, J.   (1980)   'Problematyka alkoholowa w seksuologii.'
       ['Alcohol problems in sexology.']   Problemy Alkoholizmu
       (Warsaw), 27, 7-8.

121.   GORDON, G.G., ALTMAN, K., SOUTHREN, A.L., RUBIN, E., and
       LIEBER, C.S.   (1976)   'Effect of alcohol (ethanol) admin-
       istration on sex-hormone metabolism in normal men.'
       New England Journal of Medicine, 295, 793-797.

122.   GORDON, G.G., OLIVO, J., RAFIN, F., and SOUTHREN, A.L.   (1975)
       'Conversion of androgens to estrogens in cirrhosis of the
       liver.'   Journal of Clinical Endocrinology and Metabolism,
       40, 1018-1026.

123.   GORDON, G.G., SOUTHREN, A.L., and LIEBER, C.S.   (1978)   'The
       effects of alcoholic liver disease and alcohol ingestion
       on sex hormone levels.'   Alcoholism: Clinical and Exper-
       imental Research, 2, 259-263.

124.   GORDON, G.G., SOUTHREN, A.L., and LIEBER, C.S.   (1979)   'Hypo-
       gonadism and feminization in the male: A triple effect of
       alcohol.'   [Editorial.]   Alcoholism: Clinical and Exper-
       imental Research, 3, 210-212.

125.   GORDON, G.G., VITTEK, J., HO, R., ROSENTHAL, W.S., SOUTHREN,
       A.L., and LIEBER, C.S.   (1979)   'Effect of chronic alco-
       hol use on hepatic testosterone 5-α-A-ring reductase in
       the baboon and in the human being.'   Gastroenterology, 77,
       11-114.

126.   GORDON, G.G., VITTEK, J., SOUTHREN, A.L., MUNNANGI, P., and
       LIEBER, C.S. (1980) 'Effect of chronic alcohol ingestion
       on the biosynthesis of steroids in rat testicular homo-
       genate in vitro.' Endocrinology, 106, 1880-1885.

127.   GORDON, G.G., VITTEK, J., WEINSTEIN, B., SOUTHREN, A.L., and
       LIEBER, C.S. (1979) 'Acute and chronic effects of alco-
       hol on steroid hormones with emphasis on the metabolism of
       androgens and estrogens.' In: Metabolic Effects of Alco-
       hol: Proceedings of the International Symposium on Meta-
       bolic Effects of Alcohol, Milan (June 18-21). Ed. P. Avo-
       garo, C.R. Sirtori, and E. Tremoli. Amsterdam, New York,
       and Oxford: Elsevier/North-Holland Biomedical Press,
       pp. 89-102.

128.   GORDON, G.G., WORNER, T.M., SOUTHREN, A.L., and LIEBER, C.S.
       (1981) 'Abnormal gonadotrophin releasing hormone re-
       sponses in chronically alcoholic men.' Alcoholism:
       Clinical and Experimental Research, 5, 151 (abstract).

129.   GREEN, J.R., MOWAT, N.A., and FISHER, R.A. (1976) 'Plasma
       estrogens in men with chronic liver disease.' Gut (Lon-
       don), 17, 426-430.

130.   GREENE, L.W., and HOLLANDER, C.S. (1980) 'Sex and alcohol:
       The effects of alcohol on the hypothalamic-pituitary-
       gonadal axis.' [Guest editorial.] Alcoholism: Clinical
       and Experimental Research, 4, 1-5.

131.   HAMMOND, D.C., JORGENSEN, G.Q., and RIDGEWAY, D.M. (1980)
       'Sexual adjustment of female alcoholics.' Medical As-
       pects of Human Sexuality, 14, 15.

132.   HARKONEN, M., SEUDERLING, U., ONIKKI, S., KARONEN, S.-L., and
       ADLER-CREUTZ, H. (1974) 'Low plasma testosterone values
       in men during hangover.' Journal of Steroid Biochemistry
       (Oxford), 5, 655-658.

133.   HART, B.L. (1968) 'Effects of alcohol on sexual reflexes and
       mating behavior in the male dog.' Quarterly Journal of
       Studies on Alcohol, 29, 839-844.

134.   HART, B.L. (1969) 'Effects of alcohol on sexual reflexes and
       mating behavior in the male rat.' Psychopharmacologia
       (Berlin), 14, 377-382.

135.   HAWKINS, J.L. (1976) 'Lesbianism and alcoholism.' In: Alco-
       holism Problems in Women and Children. Ed. M. Greenblatt
       and M.A. Schuckit. New York: Grune and Stratton, pp. 137-
       141.

136.   HOROWITZ, J.D., and GOBLE, A.J. (1979) 'Drugs and impaired
       male sexual function.' Drugs, 18, 206-217.

137. HUGUES, J.N., PERRET, G., ADESSI, G., COSTE, T., and MODIGLI-
     ANI, E. (1978) 'Effects of chronic alcoholism on the
     pituitary-gonadal function of women during menopausal
     transition and in the post menopausal period.' Bio-
     medicine Express (Paris), 29, 279-283.

138. HUTTUNEN, M.O., HÄRKÖNEN, M., NISKANEN, P., LEINO, T., and
     YLIKAHRI, R. (1976) 'Plasma testosterone concentrations
     in alcoholics.' Journal of Studies on Alcohol, 37, 1165-
     1177.

139. IVANOV, J. (1912) 'Der Einfluss des Alkohols auf die Sperma-
     tozen von Säugetieren und Befruchtungsversuche mit Sperma
     unter Zusatz von Alkohol.' ['The influence of alcohol on
     the spermatozoa of mammals and attempts at fertilization
     with sperms under the condition of alcohol.'] Münchener
     Medizinische Wochenschrift (Munich), 18, 998.

140. IVANOV, J. (1913) 'Action de l'alcool sur les spermatozoïdes
     des mammifères.' ['Action of alcohol on the spermatozoa
     of mammals.'] Comptes Rendus des Seances de la Societe
     de Biologie et de ses Filiales (Paris), 74, 480-482.

141. IVANOV, J. (1913) 'Expériences sur la fécondation des mammi-
     fères avec le sperme mélange d'alcool.' ['Experiences on
     the impregnation of mammals with sperm mixed with alco-
     hol.'] Comptes Rendus des Seances de la Société de Bio-
     logie et de ses Filiales (Paris), 74, 482-484.

142. JENSEN, S,B, (1981) 'Sexual dysfunction in male diabetics
     and alcoholics: A comparative study.' Sexuality and
     Disability, 4, 215-219.

143. JOHNSTON, D.E., CHIAO, Y.-B., GAVALER, J.S., and VAN THIEL,
     D.H. (1981) 'Inhibition of testosterone synthesis by
     ethanol and acetaldehyde.' Biochemical Pharmacology, 30,
     1827-1831.

144. JONES, B.M., and JONES, M.K. (1976) 'Alcohol effects in women
     during the menstrual cycle.' Annals of the New York Aca-
     demy of Sciences, 273, 576-587.

145. JONES, B.M., and JONES, M.K. (1976) 'Women and alcohol: In-
     toxication, metabolism, and the menstrual cycle.' In:
     Alcoholism Problems in Women and Children. Ed. M. Green-
     blatt and M.A. Schuckit. New York: Grune and Stratton,
     pp. 103-136.

146. JONES, M.K., TARTER, R.E., and JONES, B.M. (1981) 'The ef-
     fects of the menstrual cycle on craving in female alco-
     holics.' Alcoholism: Clinical and Experimental Research,
     5, 156 (abstract).

147. KAKIHANA, R., BUTTE, J.C., and MOORE, J.A. (1980) 'Endocrine
     effects of maternal alcoholization: Plasma and brain tes-
     tosterone dihydrotestosterone, estradiol and corticostone.'
     Alcoholism: Clinical and Experimental Research, 4, 57-61.

148. KALIN, R., MC CLELLAND, D.C., and KAHN, M. (1972) 'The ef-
     fects of male social drinking in fantasy.' In: The
     Drinking Man. Ed. D.C. Mc Clelland, W.N. Davis, R. Kalin,
     and E. Wanner. New York: The Free Press, pp. 3-20.

149. KARACAN, I., SNYDER, S., SALIS, P.J., WILLIAMS, R.L., and DER-
     MAN, S. (1980) 'Sexual dysfunction in male alcoholics
     and its objective evaluation.' In: Phenomenology and
     Treatment of Alcoholism. Ed. W.E. Fann, I. Karacan,
     A.D. Pokorny, and R.L. Williams. New York: SP Medical
     and Scientific Books, pp. 259-268.

150. KARU, E.Y. (1980) 'Po povodu stat: F.I. Stekhuna "Vliyaniye
     alkogolya na muzhskiye polovyye zhelezy."' ['Comment on
     F.I. Stekhun's paper: "Effects of alcohol on male sexual
     glands."'] Zhurnal Nevropatologie, 80, 131-132.

151. KAYUSHEVA, I.V. (1979) 'Alkogolizam i endokrinnaye sistema.'
     ['Alcohol and the endocrine system.'] Sovetskaya
     Meditsina (Moscow), 72, 87-91.

152. KENT, J.R., SCARAMUZZI, R.J., and LAUWERS, W. (1973) 'Plasma
     testosterone, estradiol and gonadotropins in hepatic in-
     sufficiency.' Gastroenterology, 64, 111-115.

153. KLASSEN, R.W., and PERSAUD, T.V.N. (1976) 'Experimental studies
     on the influence of male alcoholism on pregnancy and pro-
     geny.' Experimentelle Pathologie (Jena), 12, 38-45.

154. KLASSEN, R.W., and PERSAUD, T.V.N. (1978) 'Influence of alco-
     hol on the reproductive system of the male rat.' Inter-
     national Journal of Fertility, 23, 176-184.

155. KLASSEN, R.W., and PERSAUD, T.V.N. (1979) 'Experimental
     studies on the influence of male alcoholism on testicular
     function, pregnancy, and progeny.' Advanced Study in
     Birth Defects, 2, 239-256.

156. KLEY, H.K., STROHMEYER, G., and KRUSKEMPER, H.L. (1979) 'Ef-
     fect of testosterone application on hormone concentrations
     of androgens and estrogens in male patients with cirrhosis
     of the liver.' Gastroenterology, 76, 235-241.

157. KOSTITCH, A. (1922) 'Action de l'alcool sur les cellules sem-
     inales.' ['Alcohol action on seminal cells.'] Revue
     Internationale Contra l'Alcoolesmi, 30, 53-70.

158. KULLER, L.H., MAY, S.J., and PERPER, J.A. (1978) 'The re-
     lationship between alcohol, liver disease, and testicular
     pathology.' American Journal of Epidemiology, 108, 192-
     199.

159. KYRLE, J., and SCHOPPER, K.J. (1914) 'Untersuchungen über den
     Einfluss des Alkohols auf Liber und Hoden des Kaminchen.'
     ['Studies concerning the influence of alcohol on the liver
     and testicle of the rabbit.'] Virchows Archiv, 215, 309-
     335.

160. LANDOWSKI, J., and GILL, J. (1964) 'Einige Beobachtungen über
     das Sperma des Indischen Elefanten (Elephas maximum L.).'
     ['A few observations on the sperm of Indian elephants
     (Elephas maximum L.).'] Zoologische Garten (Leipzig),
     29, 205.

161. LANG, A.R. (1978) 'Sexual guilt, expectancies and alcohol as
     determinants of interest in and reaction to sexual stim-
     uli.' Ph.D. Dissertation, University of Wisconsin-Madi-
     son.

162. LEMERE, F., and SMITH, J.W. (1973) 'Alcohol-induced sexual
     impotence.' American Journal of Psychiatry, 130, 212-213.

163. LEPPÄLUOTO, J., RAPELI, M., VARIS, R., and RANTA, T. (1975)
     'Secretion of anterior pituitary hormones in man: Effect
     of ethyl alcohol.' Acta Physiologica Scandinavica (Stock-
     holm), 95, 400-406.

164. LESTER, R., and VAN-THIEL, D.H. (1977) 'Gonadal function in
     chronic alcoholic men.' Advances in Experimental Medicine
     and Biology, 85a, 399-414.

165. LESTER, R., and VAN-THIEL, D.H. (1977) 'Gonadal function in
     chronic alcoholic men.' In: Alcohol Intoxication and
     Withdrawal--IIIa: Biological Aspects of Ethanol.
     Ed. Milton M. Gross. New York: Plenum Press, pp. 399-
     413.

166. LEVINE, J. (1955) 'The sexual adjustment of alcoholics: A
     clinical study of a selected sample.' Quarterly Journal
     of Studies on Alcohol, 16, 675-680.

167. LIEGEL, J., FABRE, L.F., HOWARD, P.Y., and FARMER, R.W. (1972)
     'Plasma testosterone binding globulin (SBG) in alcoholic
     subjects.' Physiologist, 15, 198.

168. LINDHOLM, J., FABRICIUS-BJERRE, N., BAHNSEN, M., BOIESEN, P.,
     BANGSTRUP, L., LAU PEDERSEN, M., and HAGEN, C. (1978)
     'Pituitary-testicular function in patients with chronic
     alcoholism.' European Journal of Clinical Investigation
     (Berlin), 8, 269-272.

169. LINDHOLM, J., FABRICIUS-BJERRE, N., BAHNSEN, M., BOIESEN, P., HAGEN, C., and CHRISTENSEN, T. (1978) 'Sex steroids and sex-hormone binding globulin in males with chronic alcoholism.' European Journal of Clinical Investigation (Berlin), 8, 273-276.

170. LINNOILA, M., PRINZ, P.N., WONSOWICZ, C.J., and LEPPÄLUCTO, J. (1980) 'Effect of moderate doses of ethanol and phenobarbital on pituitary and thyroid hormones and testosterone.' British Journal of Addiction, 75, 207-212.

171. LOOSEN, P.T., and PRANGE, A.J., JR. (1977) 'Alcohol and anterior pituitary secretion.' Lancet (London), 2, 985.

172. LOX, C.D., MESSIHA, F., and HEINE, M.W. (1981) 'The influence of ethanol and oral contraceptives on reproductive physiology in the female rat.' Fertility and Sterility, 35 (Supplement), 241 (abstract).

173. LOX, C.D., MESSIHA, F.S., and HEINE, W. (1982) 'Effect of oral contraceptives on reproductive function during semi-chronic exposure to ethanol in the female rat.' General Pharmacology, 13, 53-56.

174. LOX, C.D., MESSIHA, F., HEINE, M.W., BENSON, B., and MISENHIMER, G.R. (1980) 'Ethanol and reproductive function in the female rat.' Pharmacology, Biochemistry, and Behavior, 12, 326.

175. LOX, C.D., PEDDICORD, O., HEINE, M.W., and MESSIHA, F.S. (1978) 'The influence of chronic long term alcohol abuse on testosterone secretion in men and rats.' Proceedings of the Western Pharmacology Society, 21, 299-302.

176. LYUBIMOV, B.I., SMOLNIKOVA, N.M., STREKALOVA, S.N., and YAVORSKII, A.N. (1979) ''Vliyaniye karbidina na polovyye zhelezy krys pri khronicheskom vozdeistvii etanola.' ['Effect of carbidine on the gonads of rats during chronic alcohol poisoning.] Byulleten' Eksperimental'noi Biologii Meditsiny, 87, 155-158.

177. MAC DOWELL, E.C., and LORD, E.M. (1927) 'Reproduction in alcoholic mice. I. Treated females. A study of the influence of alcohol on ovarian activity, prenatal mortality, and sex ratio.' [Wilhelm] Roux's Archives of Developmental Biology, 109, 549-581.

178. MC LACHLAN, J.A., NEWBOLD, R.R., and BULLOCK, B.C. (1980) 'Long-term effects on the female mouse genital tract associated with prenatal exposure to diethylstilbestrol.' Cancer Research, 40, 3988-3999.

179. MACMILLAN, K.L., HART, N.L., WATSON, J.D., and SMITH, J.F. (1974) 'Effects of benzyl alcohol on the bovine oestrous cycle and subsequent fertility.' Theriogenology, 1, 1-5.

180. MC NAMEE, B., GRANT, J., RATCLIFFE, J., RATCLIFFE, W. and
      OLIVER, J. (1979) 'Lack of effect of alcohol on pitui-
      tary-gonadal hormones in women.' British Journal of Addic-
      tion (Edinburgh), 74, 316-317.

181. MALATESTA, V.J. (1978) 'The effects of alcohol on ejaculation
      latency in human males.' Ph.D. Thesis, University of
      Georgia.

182. MALATESTA, V.J. POLLACK, R.H., and CROTTY, T.D. (1979) 'Alco-
      hol effects on the orgasmic response in human females.'
      Paper presented at the Annual Meeting of the Psychonomic
      Society, Phoenix, Arizona (November).

183. MALATESTA, V.J., POLLACK, R.H., WILBANKS, W.A., and ADAMS, H.E.
      (1979) 'Alcohol effects on the orgasmic-ejaculatory re-
      sponse in human males.' Journal of Sex Research, 15,
      101-107.

184. MALLOY, E.S. (1976) 'Strategies in sexual counseling in alco-
      holic marriage.' In: Sexual Counseling for Persons with
      Alcohol Problems. Ed. J. Newman. Pittsburgh, Pennsyl-
      vania: University of Pittsburgh, pp. 66-81.

185. MANDEL, L.L., and NORTH, S. (1982) 'Sex roles, sexuality, and
      the recovering woman alcoholic: Program issues.' Journal
      of Psychoactive Drugs, 14, 163-166.

186. MANN, T. (1968) 'Effects of pharmacological agents on male
      sexual functions.' Journal of Reproduction and Fertility
      (Oxford), 4 (Supplement), 101-114.

187. MARCÓ, J., LEANDRO, S.V., VILLA, I., and LARRALDE, J. (1981)
      'Efecto del etanol sobre la ovulación, reproducción y
      desarrollo fetal en la rata.' ['Effect of ethanol on ovu-
      lation, reproduction and fetal development in rats.']
      Revista Española de Fisiologia, 37, 395-402.

188. MASTERS, W.H., and JOHNSON, V.E. (1966) Human Sexual Response.
      Boston: Little, Brown, and Company, pp. 267-268.

189. MASTERS, W.H., and JOHNSON, V.E. (1970) Human Sexual In-
      adequacy. Boston: Little, Brown, and Company.

190. MEDHUS, A. (1975) 'Venereal diseases among female alcoholics.'
      Scandinavian Journal of Social Medicine, 3, 29.

191. MEDHUS, A. (1976) 'Alcohol problems among female gonorrhea
      patients.' Scandinavian Journal of Sexual Medicine, 4,
      141-143.

192. MENDELSON, J.H. (1981) 'Alcohol effects on sexual behavior
      and hormonal function.' Paper presented at the World
      Psychiatric Meeting, New York (October 31-November 1).

193. MENDELSON, J.H., ELLINGBOE, J., and MELLO, N.K. (1978) 'Ef-
     fects of alcohol on plasma testosterone and luteinizing
     hormone levels.' Alcoholism: Clinical and Experimental
     Research, 2, 255-258.

194. MENDELSON, J.H., ELLINGBOE, J., and MELLO, N.K. (1980)
     'Ethanol induced alterations in pituitary gonadal hormones
     in human males.' In: Biological Effects of Alcohol:
     Proceedings of the International Symposium on Biological
     Research in Alcoholism, Zurich, Switzerland (June, 1978).
     Ed. H. Begleiter. New York and London: Plenum Press,
     pp. 485-497.

195. MENDELSON, J.H., and MELLO, N.K. (1974) 'Alcohol, aggression,
     and androgens.' Research Publications, Association for
     Research in Nervous and Mental Disorders, 52, 225-247.

196. MENDELSON, J.H., MELLO, N.K., and ELLINGBOE, J. (1977) 'Ef-
     fects of acute alcohol intake on pituitary-gonadal hormones
     in normal human males.' Journal of Pharmacology and Ex-
     perimental Therapeutics, 202, 676-682.

197. MENDELSON, J.H., MELLO, N.K., and ELLINGBOE, J. (1978) 'Ef-
     fects of alcohol on pituitary-gonadal hormones, sexual
     function, and aggression in human males.' In: Psycho-
     pharmacology: A Generation of Progress. Ed. M.A. Lipton,
     A. DiMascio, and K.F. Killam. New York: Raven, pp. 1677-
     1692.

198. MENDELSON, J.H., MELLO, N.K., and ELLINGBOE, J. (1981) 'Acute
     alcohol intake and pituitary gonadal hormones in normal
     human females.' Journal of Pharmacology and Experimental
     Therapeutics, 218, 23-26.

199. MENENDEZ, C.E. (1980) 'Effects of alcohol on the male
     reproductive system.' In: Alcoholism: A Perspective.
     Ed. F.S. Messiha and G.S. Tyner. Westbury, New York:
     PJD Publications, pp. 69-77.

200. MERIARI, A., GINTON, A., TAMAR, H., and TOVA, L.-R. (1973)
     'Effects of alcohol on mating behavior of the female rat.'
     Quarterly Journal of Studies on Alcohol, 34, 1095-1098.

201. MOLNAR, J., and PAPP, G. (1973) 'Alkohol als möglicher
     schleimfördernder Faktor im Samen.' ['Alcohol as a
     possible stimulant of mucus production in the semen.']
     Andrologia (Berlin), 5, 105-106.

202. MONTAGUE, D.K., JAMES, R.E., JR., DE-WOLFE, V.G., and MAR-
     TIN, L.M. (1979) 'Diagnostic evaluation, classification,
     and treatment of men with sexual dysfunction.' Urology,
     14, 545-548.

203. MORGAN, M.Y., and PRATT, O.E., (1982) 'Sex, alcohol, and the
      developing fetus.' British Medical Bulletin, 38, 43-52.

204. MORRISSEY, E.R., and SCHUCKIT, M.A. (1978) 'Stressful life
      events and alcohol problems among women seen at a detox-
      ification center.' Journal of Studies on Alcohol, 39,
      1559.

205. MOŠKOVIĆ, S. (1975) 'Uticaj hronicnog trovanja alkoholom na
      ovarijunsku disfunkciju.' ['Effect of chronic alcohol in-
      toxication on ovarian dysfunction.'] Srpski Arhiv za Celo-
      kupno Lekarstvo (Belgrad), 103, 751-758.

206. MOWAT, N.A., EDWARDS, C.R., and FISHER, R. (1976) 'Hypothal-
      amic-pituitary-gonadal function in men with cirrhosis of
      the liver.' Gut (London), 17, 345-350.

207. MUNJACK, D.J. (1979) 'Sex and drugs.' Clinical Toxicology,
      15, 75-89.

208. MURPHREE, H.B. (1968) 'Addiction and sexual behavior.' In:
      Sexual Behavior and the Law. Ed. R. Slovenko. Spring-
      field, Illinois: C.C. Thomas, pp. 591-606.

209. MURPHY, W.D., COLEMAN, E., HOON, E., and SCOTT, C. (1980)
      'Sexual dysfunction and treatment in alcoholic women.'
      Sexuality and Disability, 3, 240-255.

210. NAZARYAN, S.S. (1976) 'O nekotirykh disgarmoniyakh seksual'noi
      zhizni u bol'nykh alkogolizmom.' ['Some of the disorders
      in the sex life of alcoholics.'] Zhurnal Eksperimental'noi
      i Klinicheskoi Meditsiny (Erevan), 16, 88-91.

211. NELSON, B.J. (1981) 'How alcohol affects sexually: Scientists
      investigate the paradox.' Sexual Medicine Today, 5,
      6, 7, 10, 30.

212. NELSON, J.L., OSTROWSKI, N.L., NOBLE, R.G., and REID, L.D.
      (1981) 'Naloxone reverses ethanol's effects on sexual
      behavior of the female Syrian hamster.' Physiological
      Psychology, 9, 367-370.

213. NESHKOV, N.S. (1969) 'Sostoyaniye spermatogeneza i polovoi
      funktsii u zloupotreblyayushchikh alkogolem.' ['State of
      spermatogenesis and sexual function in alcoholic abusers.']
      Vrachebnoe Delo (Kiev), 2, 130-131.

214. PARKER, F. (1959) 'Comparison of the sex temperament of alco-
      holics and moderate drinkers.' American Sociological Re-
      view, 24, 366-374.

215. PEARL, R. (1917) 'The experimental modification of germ cells.
      I. General plan of experiments with ethyl alcohol and cer-
      tain related substances.' Journal of Experimental Zoology,
      22, 125-164.

216. PEARL, R. (1917) 'The experimental modification of germ cells. II. The effect upon the domestic fowl of the daily inhalation of ethyl alcohol and certain related substances.' Journal of Experimental Zoology, 22, 165-186.

217. PEARL, R. (1917) 'The experimental modification of germ cells. III. The effect of parental alcoholism, and certain other drug intoxications, upon the progeny.' Journal of Experimental Zoology, 22, 241-310.

218. PERSKY, H., O'BRIEN, C.P., FINE, E. et al. (1977) 'The effect of alcohol and smoking on testosterone function and aggression in chronic alcoholics.' American Journal of Psychiatry, 134, 621-625.

219. PESCE, V.S. (1980) 'L'uso della droga ed i suoi riflesse sull'apparato genitale femminile.' ['The use of drugs and its effects on the female genital system.' Minerva Medica (Torino), 71, 2381-2388.

220. PHILLIPS, D.S., and STAINBROOK, G.L. (1978) 'Fecundity, natality, and weight as a function of prenatal alcohol consumption and age of the mother.' Physiological Psychology, 6, 75-77.

221. PINHAS, V. (1978) 'Sex guilt and sexual control in the woman alcoholic in early sobriety.' Unpublished doctoral dissertation, Department of Health Education, New York University.

222. PINHAS, V. (1979) 'An investigation to compare the degree to which alcoholic and non-alcoholic women report sex guilt and sexual control.' Paper presented at the National Alcoholism Forum of the National Council on Alcoholism, Washington, D.C. (April).

223. PIRON, E. (1975) 'Assessment of the male alcoholics' response to women through the use of visual stimuli.' Ph.D. dissertation, Loyola University, Chicago.

224. PODOLSKY, E. (1963) 'The woman alcoholic and premenstrual tension.' Journal of the American Medical Women's Association, 18, 816-818.

225. POTTER, J. (1979) 'Women and sex--It's enough to drive them to drink!' In: Women Who Drink: Alcoholic Experience and Psychotherapy. Ed. V. Burtle. Springfield, Illinois: Charles C. Thomas.

226. POWELL, B.J., VIAMONTES, J.A., and BROWN, C.S. (1974) 'Alcohol effects on the sexual potency of alcoholic and non-alcoholic males.' Alcoholism (Zagreb), 10, 78-80.

227. POWELL, D.J. (1980) 'Sexual dysfunction and alcoholism.' Journal of Sex Education and Therapy, 6, 40-46.

228. RACHAMIN, G., MAC DONALD, J.A., WAHID, S., CLAPP, J.J., KHANNA,
      J.M., and ISRAEL, Y. (1980) 'Modulation of alcohol dehy-
      drogenase and ethanol metabolism by sex hormones in the
      spontaneously hypertensive rat.' Biochemical Journal, 186,
      483-490.

229. RAMAN, G., PURANDARE, T.V., and MUNSHI, S.R. (1976) 'Steril-
      ity induced in male rats by injection of chemical agents
      into the vas deferens.' Andrologia, 8, 321-325.

230. REDMOND, G.P. (1980) 'Effect of ethanol on pulsatile gonado-
      tropin secretion in the male rat.' Alcoholism: Clinical
      and Experimental Research, 4, 226 (abstract).

231. ROSENFELD, G. (1905) 'Alkohol und Geschlechtsleben.' ['Alco-
      hol and sex life.'] Zeitschrift für Bekämpfung der
      Geschlechtskrankheiten, 3, 321-335.

232. ROWE, P.H., RACEY, P.A., and SHENTON, J.C., ELLWOOD, M., and
      LEHANE, J. (1974) 'Effects of acute administration of
      alcohol and barbiturates on plasma luteinizing hormone and
      testosterone in man.' Journal of Endocrinology (London),
      63, 50P-51P (abstract).

233. RUBIN, E., LIEBER, C.S., ALTMAN, K., GORDON, G.G., and SOUTH-
      ERN, A.L. (1976) 'Prolonged ethanol consumption in-
      creases testosterone metabolism in the liver.' Science,
      191, 563-564.

234. RUBIN, H.B., and HENSON, D.E. (1976) 'Effects of alcohol on
      male sexual responding.' Psychopharmacology (Berlin),
      47, 123-134.

235. RYBACK, R.S. (1977) 'Chronic alcohol consumption and menstru-
      ation.' [Letter.] Journal of the American Medical Assoc-
      iation, 238, 2143.

236. SAGHIR, M.T., ROBINS, E., WALBRAN, B., and GENTRY, K.A. (1970)
      'Homosexuality. IV. Psychiatric disorders and disability
      in the female homosexual.' American Journal of Psychiatry,
      127, 147-154.

237. SAUL, G. (1959) 'Blockade of ovulation in the rabbit by in-
      toxicating doses of ethyl alcohol.' Anatomical Record,
      133, 332 (abstract).

238. SCHAPOSNIK, F., SALVIOLI, M.V., CAPUTO, C.H., and CASTELLETO, R.
      (1978) 'Alteraciones histopatológicas testiculares en el
      alcoholismo crónico.' ['Testicular histopathological
      changes in chronic alcoholism.'] Revista Clinica Españo-
      la, 150, 35-38.

239. SCHEID, R. (1975) 'Changes in sexual performance due to liver
      disease.' Medical Aspects of Human Sexuality, 19, 67-79.

240. SCHEIG, R. (1982) 'Effect of alcohol on testosterone.'
      Medical Aspects of Human Sexuality, 16, 179-180.

241. SCHUCKIT, M.A. (1972) 'Sexual disturbance in the woman alco-
      holic.' Medical Aspects of Human Sexuality, 6, 44-62.

242. SCHUSTER, R. (1980) 'Zur (sexuellen) Hemmungsfähigkeit bei
      niedriger Blutalkoholkonzentration: Eine experimentelle
      Untersuchung.' ['Sexual inhibition at low blood alcohol
      concentrations: An experimental study.'] Beiträge zur
      Gerichtlichen Medizin, 38, 337-342.

243. SEMCZUK, M. (1978) 'Further investigations on the ultra-
      structure of spermatozoa in chronic alcoholics.' Zeit-
      schrift für Mikroskopisch-Anatomische Forschung, 92,
      494-508.

244. SEMCZUK, M. (1978) 'Morphological research on the male gonad
      in long-lasting alcoholization of rats.' Gegenbaurs Mor-
      phologisches Jahrbuch, 124, 546-558.

245. SEMCZUK, M. (1978) 'Ocena plemnikow szczurow poddanych przew-
      lekłej intoksykacji alkoholem etylowym.' ['Evaluation of
      rat sperm following chronic alcohol intoxication.']
      Ginekologia Polska, 49, 955-961.

246. SEMCZUK, M. (1979) '3-beta-hydroxysteroid dehydrogenase
      activity and the morphological structure of Leydig's cells
      in white rat testicles under conditions of longlasting
      alcohol intoxication.' Materia Medica Polona, 11, 132-
      138.

247. SEMCZUK, M., MAJEWSKA, T., and JACH, E. (1980) 'Wptyw in-
      toksykacji alkoholowej na stan morfologiczny najadrza
      szczura białego po podaniu estrogenów, testosteronu i
      gonadotropiny.' ['Effect of alcohol intoxication on the
      morphology of albino rat epididymus after administration
      of estrogens, testosterone, and gonadotropin.']
      Ginekologia Polska, 51, 1063-1071.

248. SEMCZUK, M., ŹRUBEK, H., and CZAJKA, R. (1978) 'Dalsze badania
      nad morfologią nasienia mężczyzn dotknietych przewlekłym
      alkoholizmem.' ['Morphology of sperm in chronic alco-
      holics.'] Polski Tygodnik Lekarski (Warsaw), 33, 961-964.

249. SHARMA, S.C., and CHAUDHURY, R.R. (1970) 'Studies on mating.
      Part II: The effect of ethanol on sperm transport and
      ovulation in successfully mated rabbits.' Indian Journal
      of Medical Research (New Delhi), 58, 501-504.

250. SHOLTY, M.J. (1979) 'Female sexual experience and satis-
      faction as related to alcohol consumption.' Unpublished
      manuscript. Alcohol and Drug Abuse Program, University
      of Maryland at Baltimore.

251. SIMIONESCU, L., OPRESCU, M., PROTICI, M., and DIMITRIU, V.
          (1977) 'The hormonal pattern in alcoholic disease.
          I. Luteinizing hormone (LH), follicle-stimulating hormone
          (TSH), and testosterone.' Endokrinologie, 15, 45.

252. SIMMONDS, H. (1898) 'Über die Ursache der Azoospermie.' ['On
          the cause of inability to produce spermatozoa.'] Inter-
          nationale Monatsschrift, 8, 383.

253. SIMMONDS, K. (1898) 'Über die Ursachen der Azoospermie.' ['On
          the causes of inability to produce spermatozoa.'] Berliner
          Klinische Wochenschrift (Berlin), 36, 806.

254. SMITH, J.W. (1972) 'Impotence in alcoholism.' Northwestern
          Medicine, 71, 523-524.

255. SOUTHREN, A.L., and GORDON, G.G. (1970) 'Studies in androgen
          metabolism.' Mount Sinai Journal of Medicine, 37, 516-527.

256. SOUTHREN, A.L., and GORDON, G.G. (1976) 'Effects of alcohol
          and alcoholic cirrhosis on sex hormone metabolism.'
          Fertility and Sterility, 27, 202-206.

257. SOUTHREN, A.L., GORDON, G.G., OLIVO, J., ROSENTHAL, W.S., and
          RAFII, F. (1973) 'Androgen metabolism in cirrhosis of the
          liver.' Metabolism, 22, 695-702.

258. SOUTHREN, A.L., GORDON, G.G., and TOCHIMOTO, S. (1968) 'Fur-
          ther study of factors affecting the metabolic clearance
          rate of testosterone in man.' Journal of Clinical Endo-
          crinology and Metabolism, 28, 1108-1112.

259. SPARROW, D., BOSSE, R., and ROWE, J.W. (1980) 'The influence
          of age, alcohol consumption, and body build on gonadal
          function in men.' Journal of Clinical Endocrinology and
          Metabolism, 51, 508-512.

260. STEKHUN, F.I. (1979) 'Alkogol i tabakokureniye kak vozmozhnyye
          prichiny besplodiya muzhchin.' ['Alcohol and tobacco
          smoking as possible causes of sterility in men.'] Vestn.
          Derm. Vener., No. 7, 61-65.

261. STEKHUN, F.I. (1979) 'Vliyaniye alkogolya na muzhskiye polovye
          zhelezy.' ['Influence of alcohol on the male sexual
          glands.'] Zhurnal Nevropatologii i Psikhiatrii Imeni s s
          Korsakova (Moscow), 79, 192-195.

262. STOKES, P.E. (1971) 'Alcohol-endocrine interrelationships.'
          In: The Biology of Alcoholism. Volume 1: Biochemistry.
          Ed. B. Kissin and H. Begleiter. New York: Plenum Press.

263. SUNDAR, P.S., SIALY, R., and DASH, R.J. (1981) 'Bardet biedl
          syndrome: A case report with special reference to studies
          on hypothalamo-pituitary testicular axis.' Journal of
          Associated Physicians of India, 29, 485-487.

264. SYMONS, A.M., and MARKS, V. (1975) 'The effects of alcohol on
      weight gain and the hypothalamic-pituitary-gonadotrophin
      axis in the maturing male rat.' Biochemical Pharmacology,
      24, 955-958.

265. TEITELBAUM, H.A., and GANTT, W.H. (1958) 'The effect of alcohol
      on sexual reflexes and sperm count in the dog.' Quarterly
      Journal of Studies on Alcohol, 19, 394-398.

266. THORNER, M.O., KIRK, C.R., and MAC LEOD, R.M. (1978) 'Alcohol
      stimulation of prolactin release from perfused isolated
      rat pituitary cells.' Federation Proceedings, 37, 637
      (abstract).

267. TODD, W.H. (1973) 'Truth about sex and alcohol.' Memorial
      Mercury, 13, 15-16.

268. TROXELL, S., JACOBSON, S., SEHGAL, P., and BURNAP, J. (1981)
      'Decreased fertility as a consequence of chronic ethanol
      consumption in the monkey.' Alcoholism: Clinical and
      Experimental Research, 5, 170 (abstract).

269. VAN THIEL, D.H. (1979) 'Feminization of chronic alcoholic
      men: A formulation.' Yale Journal of Biology and
      Medicine, 52, 219-225.

270. VAN THIEL, D.H. (1981) 'Ethanol and pituitary gonadal hor-
      mones.' Alcoholism: Clinical and Experimental Research,
      5, 577-578.

271. VAN THIEL, D.H. (1981) 'Hypothalamic-pituitary-gonadal func-
      tion in liver disease.' Progress in Biochemical Pharma-
      cology. Volume 18: Endocrinological Aspects of Alco-
      holism. Ed. F.S. Messiha and G.S. Tyner. Basel, Switzer-
      land: S. Karger, 24-34.

272. VAN THIEL, D.H. (1982) 'An introduction.' Alcoholism: Clin-
      ical and Experimental Research, 6, 178.

273. VAN THIEL, D.C., BALABAUD, C., MAGNE, F., SARIC, J., and
      BIOULAC, P. (1981) 'Alcohol and hypogonadism.' Gastro-
      enterology, 80, 882.

274. VAN THIEL, D.H., and GAVALER, J.S. (1982) 'The adverse effects
      of ethanol upon hypothalamic-pituitary-gonadal function in
      males and females compared and contrasted.' Alcoholism:
      Clinical and Experimental Research, 6, 179-185.

275. VAN THIEL, D.H., GAVALER, J.S., COBB, C.F., SHERINS, R.J., and
      LESTER, R. (1979) 'Alcohol-induced testicular atrophy in
      the adult male rat.' Endocrinology, 105, 888-895.

276. VAN THIEL, D.H., GAVALER, J.S., EAGON, P.K., CHIAO, Y.-B.,
      COBB, C.F., and LESTER, R. (1980) 'Alcohol and sexual
      function.' Pharmacology, Biochemistry, and Behavior, 13,
      Supplement 1, 125-129.

277. VAN THIEL, D.H., GAVALER, J.S., EAGON, P.K., CHIAO, Y-B., and
      LESTER, R. (1981) 'Hypogonadism and feminization in
      alcoholic men: The past, present, and future.' Currents
      in Alcoholism, 8, 29-40.

278. VAN THIEL, D.II., GAVALER, J.S., EAGON, P.L., COBB, C.F.,
      CHIAO, Y.-B., and LESTER, R. (1981) 'Adverse effects of
      ethanol upon sexual functioning: Experimental studies in
      animals.' Currents in Alcoholism, 8, 471-477.

279. VAN THIEL, D.H., GAVALER, J.S., HERMAN, G.B., LESTER, R.,
      SMITH, W.I., JR., and GAY, V.L. (1980) 'An evaluation
      of the respective roles of liver disease and malnutrition
      in the pathogenesis of the hypogonadism seen in alcoholic
      rats.' Gastroenterology, 79, 533-538.

280. VAN THIEL, D.H., GAVALER, J.S., and LESTER, R. (1974) 'Eth-
      anol inhibition of vitamin A metabolism in the testes:
      Possible mechanism for sterility in alcoholics.' Science,
      186, 941-942.

281. VAN THIEL, D.H., GAVALER, J.S., and LESTER, R. (1977) 'Eth-
      anol: A gonadal toxin in the female.' Drug and Alcohol
      Dependence (Lausanne), 2, 373-380.

282. VAN THIEL, D.H., GAVALER, J.S., and LESTER, R. (1978) 'Alco-
      hol-induced ovarian failure in the rat.' Journal of
      Clinical Investigation, 61, 624-632.

283. VAN THIEL, D.H., GAVALER, J.S., LESTER, R., and GOODMAN, M.D.
      (1975) 'Alcohol-induced testicular atrophy: An exper-
      imental model for hypogonadism occurring in chronic alco-
      holic men.' Gastroenterology, 69, 326-332.

284. VAN THIEL, D.H., GAVALER, J.S., LESTER, R., LORIAUX, D.L., and
      BRAUNSTEIN, G.D. (1975) 'Plasma estrone, prolactin,
      neurophysin, and sex steroid-binding globulin in chronic
      alcoholic men.' Metabolism: Clinical and Experimental,
      24, 1015-1019.

285. VAN THIEL, D.H., GAVALER, J.S., LESTER, R., and SHERINS, R.J.
      (1978) 'Alcohol-induced ovarian failure in the rat.'
      Journal of Clinical Investigation, 61, 624-632.

286. VAN THIEL, D.H., GAVALER, J.S., SLONE, F.L., COBB, C.F.,
      SMITH, W.I., JR., BRON, K.M., and LESTER, R. (1980) 'Is
      feminization in alcoholic men due in part to portal hyper-
      tension: A rat model.' Gastroenterology, 78, 81-91.

287. VAN THIEL, D.H., and LESTER, R. (1974) 'Sex and alcohol.'
      New England Journal of Medicine, 291, 251-253.

288. VAN THIEL, D.H., and LESTER, R. (1976) 'Alcoholism: Its ef-
      fect on hypothalamic-pituitary-gonadal function.' Gastro-
      enterology, 71, 318-327.

289. VAN THIEL, D.H., and LESTER, R. (1976) 'Sex and alcohol: A
      second peek.' New England Journal of Medicine, 295, 826-
      835.

290. VAN THIEL, D.H., and LESTER, R. (1979) 'The effect of chronic
      alcohol abuse on sexual function.' Clinics in Endocrin-
      ology and Metabolism, 8, 499-510.

291. VAN THIEL, D.H., LESTER, R., and SHERINS, R.J. (1974) 'Hypo-
      gonadism in alcoholic liver disease: Evidence for a
      double defect.' Gastroenterology, 67, 1188-1199.

292. VAN THIEL, D.H., LESTER, R., and VAITUKAITIS, J. (1978) 'Evi-
      dence for a defect in pituitary secretion of luteinizing
      hormone in chronic alcoholic men.' Journal of Clinical
      Endocrinology and Metabolism, 47, 499-507.

293. VAN THIEL, D.H., and LORIAUX, D.L. (1979) 'Evidence for an
      adrenal origin of plasma estrogens in alcoholic men.'
      Metabolism: Clinical and Experimental, 28, 536-541.

294. VAN THIEL, D.H., MC CLAIN, C.J., ELSON, M.K., MC MILLAN, M.J.,
      and LESTER, R. (1978) 'Evidence for autonomous secretion
      of prolactin in some alcoholic men with cirrhosis and
      gynecomastia.' Metabolism: Clinical and Experimental,
      27, 1778-1784.

295. VITÉZ, M., and CZEIZEL, E. (1982) 'Az iszákos-alkoholista nők
      termékenysege.' ['Fecundity of female alcoholics.']
      Alkohólogia (Budapest), 13, 79-83.

296. WEATHERSBEE, P.S., and LODGE, J.R. (1978) 'A review of eth-
      anol's effects on the reproductive process.' Journal of
      Reproductive Medicine, 21, 63-78.

297. WEDECK, H.E. (1961) Dictionary of Aphrodisiacs. New York:
      Philosophical Library.

298. WEICHSELBAUM, A., and KYRLE, J. (1911) 'Über die Veranderer-
      ungen der Hoden bei chronischem Alkoholismus.' ['On the
      changes in the testicles in chronic alcoholism.'] Sitz-
      ungsberichte der Akademie der Wissenschaften in Wien
      (Mathematischnaturwissenschaftliche Klasse), 120, 56-66.

299. WELLER, C.V. (1916) 'Histological studies of the testes of
      guinea pigs showing lead blastophthoria.' Proceedings
      of the Society for Experimental Biology and Medicine,
      14, 14.

300. WELLER, C.V.   (1921)   'Testicular changes in acute alcoholism
        in man and their relationship to blastophthoria.'   Pro-
        ceedings of the Society for Experimental Biology, 19,
        131-132.

301. WELLER, C.V.   (1930)   'Degenerative changes in the male ger-
        minal epithelium in acute alcoholism and their possible
        relationship to blastophthoria.'   American Journal of
        Pathology, 6, 1-18.

302. WESTLING, A.   (1954)   'On the correlation of the consumption
        of alcoholic drinks with some sexual phenomenon of Finnish
        male students.'   International Journal of Sexology, 7,
        109-115.

303. WHALLEY, L.J.   (1978)   'Sexual adjustment of male alcoholics.'
        Acta Psychiatrica Scandinavica (Copenhagen), 58, 281-298.

304. WHALLEY, L.J., and MC GUIRE, R.J.   (1978)   'Measuring sexual
        attitudes.'   Acta Psychiatrica Scandinavica (Copenhagen),
        58, 299-314.

305. WILLIAMS, K.H.   (1976)   'An overview of sexual problems in alco-
        holism.'   In: Sexual Counseling for Persons with Alcohol
        Problems: Proceedings of a Workshop.   Ed. J. Newman.   Wes-
        tern Pennsylvania Institute of Alcohol Studies, University
        of Pittsburgh, pp. 1-23.

306. WILMOT, R.   (1981)   'Sexual drinking and drift.'   Journal of
        Drug Issues (Winter), 1-16.

307. WILSNACK, S.C.   (1973)   'Sex role identity in female alco-
        holism.'   Journal of Abnormal Psychology, 82, 253-261.

308. WILSNACK, S.C.   (1974)   'The effects of social drinking on
        women's fantasy.'   Journal of Personality, 42, 43-61.

309. WILSNACK, S.C.   (1976)   'The impact of sex roles on women's
        alcohol use and abuse.'   In: Alcoholism Problems in
        Women and Children.   Ed. M. Greenblatt and M.A. Schuckit.
        New York: Grune and Stratton, pp. 37-63.

310. WILSNACK, S.C.   (1981)   'Alcohol, sexuality, and reproductive
        dysfunction in women.'   In: Fetal Alcohol Syndrome.
        Volume 2:   Human Studies.   Ed. E.L. Abel.   Boca Raton,
        Florida: CRC Press.

311. WILSNACK, S.C., and WILSNACK, R.W.   (1979)   'Sex roles and
        adolescent drinking.'   In: Youth, Alcohol, and Social
        Policy.   Ed. H.T. Blane and M.E. Chafetz.   New York:
        Plenum Press, pp. 183-227.

312. WILSON, G.T.   (1977)   'Alcohol and human sexual behavior.'   Be-
        havior Research and Therapy (Oxford), 15, 239-252.

313. WILSON, G.T., and LAWSON, D.M.   (1976) 'Effects of alcohol on
      sexual arousal in women.' Journal of Abnormal Psychology,
      85, 489-497.

314. WILSON, G.T., and LAWSON, D.M.   (1976) 'Expectancies, alcohol,
      and sexual arousal in male social drinkers.' Journal of
      Abnormal Psychology, 85, 587-594.

315. WILSON, G.T., and LAWSON, D.M.   (1978) 'Expectancies, alcohol,
      and sexual arousal in women.' Journal of Abnormal Psy-
      chology, 87, 358-367.

316. WILSON, G.T., LAWSON, D.M., and ABRAMS, D.B.   (1978) 'Effects
      of alcohol on sexual arousal in male alcoholics.' Journal
      of Abnormal Psychology, 87, 609-616.

317. WRIGHT, J.W., FRY, D.E., MERRY, J., and MARKS, V.   (1976)
      'Abnormal hypothalamic-pituitary-gonadal function in
      chronic alcoholics.' British Journal of Addiction (Edin-
      burgh), 71, 211-215.

318. WRIGHT, J., MERRY, J., FRY, J., and MARKS, V.   (1975) 'Pit-
      uitary function in chronic alcoholism.' Advanced Exper-
      iments in Medical Biology, 59, 253.

319. YESSIAN, N., and NOBLE, E.P.   (1981) 'In vitro testosterone
      synthesis by rat testes following chronic alcohol admin-
      istration.' Federation Proceedings, 40, 825 (abstract).

320. YLIKAHRI, R.H.   (1978) 'Acute effects of alcohol on anterior
      pituitary secretion of tropic hormones.' Clinical Endo-
      crinology and Metabolism, 46, 715-720.

321. YLIKAHRI, R.H., HUTTUNEN, M.O., and HÄRKÖNEN, M.   (1980)
      'Hormonal changes during alcohol intoxication and with-
      drawal.' Pharmacology, Biochemistry, and Behavior, 13,
      131-137.

322. YLIKAHRI, R.H., HUTTUNEN, M.O., HÄRKÖNEN, M., SEUDERLING, U.,
      ONIKKI, S., KARONEN, S.-L., and ADLERCREUTZ, H.   (1974)
      'Low plasma testosterone values in men during hangover.'
      Journal of Steroid Biochemistry (Oxford), 5, 655-658.

Amphetamines

323. ABBATIELLO, E.R., and DALY, I. (1975) 'Effects of D-amphetamine sulfate on aggressive behavior in laboratory mice.' Clinical Toxicology, 8, 337-347.

324. ALPERN, E.B., FINKELSTEIN, N., and GANTT, W.H. (1941) 'Effect of amphetamine sulfate on the nervous activity of dogs.' American Journal of Physiology, 133, 196.

325. ANDY, C.J. (1977) 'Hypersexuality and limbic system seizures.' Pavlovian Journal of Biological Science, 12, 187-228.

326. ANGRIST, B., and GERSHON, S. (1972) 'Psychiatric sequelae of amphetamine abuse.' In: R.I. Shaden, ed. Psychiatric Complications of Medical Drugs. New York: Raven Press.

327. ANGRIST, B., and GERSHON, S. (1972) 'Some recent studies on amphetamine psychosis--unresolved issues.' In: E.H. Ellinwood and S. Cohen, eds. Current Concepts on Amphetamine Abuse. Proceedings of a Workshop, Duke University Medical Center, June 5-6, 1970. Washington, D.C.: U.S. Government Printing Office, pp. 193-204.

328. ANGRIST, B., and GERSHON, S. (1976) 'Clinical effects of amphetamine and L-dopa on sexuality and aggression.' Comprehensive Psychiatry, 17, 715-722.

329. BEATTY, W.W., DODGE, A.M., and TRAYLOR, K.L. (1982) 'Stereotyped behavior elicited by amphetamine in the rat: Influences of the testes.' Pharmacology, Biochemistry, and Behavior, 16, 565-568.

330. BECKER, J.B., ROBINSON, T.E., and LORENZ, K.A. (1982) 'Sex differences and estrous cycle variations in amphetamine-elicited rotational behavior.' European Journal of Pharmacology, 80, 65-72.

331.   BELL, D.S., and TRETHOWAN, W.H.   (1961)   'Amphetamine addiction.'
        Journal of Nervous and Mental Diseases, 133, 491-492.

332.   BELL, D.S., and TRETHOWAN, W.H.   (1961)   'Amphetamine addiction
        and disturbed sexuality.'   Archives of General Psychiatry,
        4, 474-478.

333.   BERMAN, L.E.A.   (1972)   'The role of amphetamine in a case of
        hysteria.'   Journal of the American Psychoanalytical Assoc-
        iation, 20, 329.

334.   BETT, W.R.   (1946)   'Benzedrine sulfate in clinical medicine:
        A survey of the literature.'   Postgraduate Medical Journal,
        22, 205-218.

335.   BIGNAMI, C.   (1966)   'Pharmacological influence on mating behavior
        in the male rat: Effect of D-amphetamine, LSD-25, strych-
        nine, nicotine, and various anticholinergic agents.'   Psycho-
        pharmacologia, 10, 44.

336.   BINDEMANN, S., WELLS, B.W., FISH, F., and SCHOFIELD, C.B.   (1976)
        'Drug misuse in a special clinic patient population in
        Glasgow.'   British Journal of Venereal Diseases, 52, 343-
        347.

337.   BONHOFF, G., and LEWRENZ, H.   (1954)   Über Weckamine (Perritin
        und Benzedrin).   [On Stimulants (Perritin and Benzedrine).]
        Berlin, Göttingen, and Heidelberg: Springer-Verlag.

338.   BROITMAN, S.T., and DONOSO, A.O.   (1975)   'Modifications of post-
        coital LH secretion and oestrous behaviour induced by drugs
        in ovariectomized rats.'   Journal of Reproduction and Fer-
        tility, 44, 309-312.

339.   BUTCHER, L.L., BUTCHER, S.G., and LARSSON, K.   (1969)   'Effects
        of apomorphine(+)-amphetamine, and nialamide on tetraben-
        azine-induced suppression of sexual behavior in the male
        rat.'   European Journal of Pharmacology, 7, 283-288.

340.   CAREY, J.T., and MANDEL, J.   (1968)   'A San Francisco Bay area
        "speed" scene.'   Journal of Health and Social Behavior, 9,
        164-174.

341.   CARR, R.B.   (1954)   'Acute psychotic reaction after inhaling
        methylamphetamine.'   British Medical Journal, 1, 1976.

342.   CARTER, C.S., BAHR, J.M., and RAMIREZ, V.D.   (1978)   'Monoamines,
        estrogen, and female sexual behavior in the golden hamster.'
        Brain Research, 144, 109-121.

343.   COHEN, M., and KLEIN, D.F.   (1972)   'Age of onset of drug abuse
        in psychiatric inpatients.'   Archives of General Psychiatry,
        26, 266-269.

344.   COHEN, M., and KLEIN, D.F.   (1970)   'Drug abuse in a young psy-
       chiatric population.' American Journal of Orthopsychiatry,
       40, 448-455.

345.   CONNELL, P.H. (1958) Amphetamine Psychosis. Maudsley Mono-
       graph No. 5. London: Oxford University Press.

346.   COX, C., and SMART, R.G. (1972) 'Social and psychological
       aspects of speed use: A study of types of speed users in
       Toronto.' International Journal of the Addictions, 7,
       201-217.

347.   COX, C., and SMART, R.G. (1970) 'The nature and extent of
       speed use in North America.' Canadian Medical Association
       Journal, 102, 724-729.

348.   CREMIEUX, A., CAIN, J., and RABATTU, J. (1948) 'Toxicomanie
       alcoolique et ortedrine chez un desequilibre de la sexualité.'
       ['Addiction to alcohol and amphetamine in a sexual pervert.']
       Annales Médico-Psychologiques, 106, 497-501.

349.   DAHLBERG, C.C. (1971) 'Sexual behavior in the drug culture.'
       Medical Aspects of Human Sexuality, 5, 64-71.

350.   DALLO, J., and HELD, K. (1972) 'Drugs and sexual behaviour in
       rats.' Activitas Nervosa Superior, 14, 303.

351.   DOEPFMER, R. (1966) 'Therapy with psychopharmaca in functional
       disorders of the male genitalia.' [In German.] Hippokrates,
       37, 298-301.

352.   DONOSO, A.O. (1977) 'Blockage of progesterone-induced release of
       luteinizing hormone and prolactin by D-amphetamine and fen-
       fluramine in rats.' Psychopharmacology, 55, 173-176.

353.   EARLEY, C.J., and LEONARD, E.E. (1978) 'Behavioural studies
       on the effects of D-amphetamine and estradiol benzoate
       alone and in combination.' Psychopharmacology, 56, 179-183.

354.   ELIASSON, M., MICHANEK, A., and MEYERSSON, B.J. (1972) 'A
       differential inhibitory action of LSD and amphetamine on
       copulatory behaviour in the female rat.' In: Animal Pharm.
       Uppsala: Uppsala University Biomedical Center (22 pp.).

355.   ELLINWOOD, E.H. (1967) 'Amphetamine psychosis. I. Description
       of the individuals and process.' Journal of Nervous and
       Mental Diseases, 144, 273-283.

356.   ELLINWOOD, E.H. (1969) 'Amphetamine psychosis: A multidimen-
       sional process.' Seminars in Psychiatry, 1, 208-226.

357.   ELLINWOOD, E.H. (1972) 'Amphetamine psychosis: Individuals, settings, and sequences.' In: E.H. Ellinwood and S. Cohen, eds. Current Concepts on Amphetamine Abuse. Washington, D.C.: U.S. Government Printing Office, pp. 143-158.

358.   ELLINWOOD, E.H., and ROCKWELL, W.J.K. (1975) 'Effect of drug use on sexual behavior.' Medical Aspects of Human Sexuality, 9, 10-32.

359.   FERGUSON, J., and DEMENT, W. (1969) 'The behavioral effects of amphetamine on REM deprived rats.' Journal of Psychiatric Research, 7, 111-118.

360.   FIDDLE, S. (1968) 'The case of "peak user" John.' In: J.R. Russo, ed. Amphetamine Abuse. Springfield, Illinois: C.C. Thomas, pp. 119-146.

361.   FLORIO, V., FUENTES, J.A., ZIEGLER, H., and LONGO, V.G. (1972) 'EEG and behavioral effects in animals of some amphetamine derivatives with hallucinogenic properties.' Behavioral Biology, 7, 401-414.

362.   FROMMEL, E., SEYDOUX, J., VON LEDEBUR, I., CHMOULIOVSKY, M., and PRASAD, C.R. (1966) 'Neuropharmacological study of central reactions to intense muscular exertion, sensorial fatigue, sexual excitation, hunger, and thirst.' Medicina et Pharmacologia Experimentalis, 14 (Supplement), 1-56.

363.   GAWIN, F.H. (1978) 'Pharmacologic enhancement of the erotic: Implications of an expanded definition of aphrodisiacs.' Journal of Sex Research, 14, 107-117.

364.   GAY, G.R., NEWMEYER, J., ELION, R., and WIEDER, S. (1975) 'Drug/sex practice in the Haight-Ashbury or "the sensuous hippie."' In: National Academy of Sciences. Problems of Drug Dependence, 1975: Proceedings of the 37th Annual Scientific Meeting. Committee on Problems of Drug Dependence. Washington, D.C.: The Academy, pp. 1080-1093.

365.   GAY, G.R., and SHEPPARD, C.W. (1972) 'Sex in the "drug culture."' Medical Aspects of Human Sexuality, 6, 28-47.

366.   GAY, G.R., and SHEPPARD, C.W. (1973) 'Sex-crazed dope fiends--mth or reality.' Drug Forum, 2, 125-140.

367.   GAY, G.R., and SHEPPARD, C.W. (1973) 'Sex-crazed dope fiends! Myth or reality.' In: E. Harms, ed. Drugs and Youth: The Challenge of Today. New York: Pergamon Press, pp. 149-163.

368.   GEERLINGS, P. (1972) 'Social and psychiatric factors in amphetamine users.' Psychiatria, Neurologica, Neurochirurgia, 75, 219-224.

369.   GOLDBERG, L. (1968) 'Drug abuse in Sweden.' Bulletin on Narcotics, 20, 1.

370.   GONZALEZ-BARÓN, S., JIMÉNEZ-VARGAS, J., and LOPEZ, G.G. (1971)
        'Cambios en el ciclo ovarico por anfetamina y reserpina.'
        ['Changes in the ovarian cycle caused by amphetamine and
        reserpine.'] Revista de Medicina de la Universidad de
        Navarra, 15, 251-259.

371.   GOSSOP, M., STERN, R., and CONNELL, P. (1974) 'Drug dependence
        and sexual dysfunction: A comparison of intravenous users
        of narcotics and oral use of amphetamines.' British Journal
        of Psychiatry, 124, 431-434.

372.   GREAVES, G. (1972) 'Sexual disturbances among chronic amphet-
        amine users.' Journal of Nervous and Mental Diseases, 155,
        363-365.

373.   GRIFFITH, J. (1966) 'A study of illicit amphetamine drug traf-
        fic in Oklahoma City.' American Journal of Psychiatry, 123,
        560-569.

374.   GRINSPOON, L., and HEDBLOM, P. (1975) The Speed Culture: Am-
        phetamine Use and Abuse in America. Cambridge, Massachu-
        setts: Harvard University Press.

375.   GUTTMANN, E. (1939) 'Discussion on benzedrine: Uses and
        abuses.' Proceedings of the Royal Society of Medicine,
        32, 389.

376.   HALBREICH, U., SACHAR, E.J., ASNIS, G.M., NATHAN, R.S., and
        HALPERN, F.S. (1981) 'The prolactin response to intra-
        venous dextroamphetamine in normal young men and postmeno-
        pausal women.' Life Sciences, 28, 2337-2342.

377.   HAMPTON, W.H. (1961) 'Observed psychiatric reactions following
        use of amphetamine and amphetamine-like substances.'
        Bulletin of the New York Academy of Medicine, 37, 172.

378.   HARDER, A. (1947) 'Über Weckamin-Psychoses.' ['On wake-amine
        psychoses.'] Schweizerische Medizinische Wochenschrift, 77,
        982-985.

379.   HAWKS, D., MITCHESON, M., OGBORNE, A., and EDWARDS, G. (1969)
        'Abuse of methylamphetamine.' British Medical Journal, 2,
        715-720.

380.   HENSLER, J.M. (1970) 'Changes in perceptions of sexual exper-
        iences of college students while under the influence of
        drugs.' Committee on Problems of Drug Dependence, p. 6531.

381.   HERNDON, J.G., and NEILL, D.B. (1973) 'Amphetamine reversal of
        sexual impairment following anterior hypothalamic lesions in
        female rats.' Pharmacology, Biochemistry, and Behavior, 1,
        285-288.

382. HERZ, S. (1968) 'Behavioral patterns in sex and drug use on
      three campuses: Implications for education and society.'
      Psychiatric Quarterly, 42, 258-271.

383. HERZ, S. (1970) 'Behavioral patterns in sex and drug use on the
      college campus.' Journal of the Medical Society of New Jer-
      sey, 67, 3-6.

384. ISBELL, H. (1969) 'General aspects of the treatment of drug
      dependence relevant to the abuse of amphetamines and amphet-
      amine-like compounds.' In: F. Sjoqvist and M. ToHie, eds.
      Abuse of Central Stimulants. Stockholm: Almqvist and Wik-
      sell, pp. 15-30.

385. JACKSON, B., and REED, A. (1970) 'Another abusable amphetamine.'
      Journal of the American Medical Association, 211, 830.

386. JIMÉNEZ-VARGAS, J., GONZALEZ-BARÓN, S., and HERNANDEZ, F. (1973)
      'Effects of amphetamine and reserpine on ovulation: Quanti-
      tative study.' [In Spanish.] Revista de Medicina de la
      Universidad de Navarra, 17, 1-8.

387. JONES, H.B. (1974) 'The effects of sensual drugs on behavior:
      Clues to the function of the brain.' Advances in Psycho-
      biology, 2, 297-312.

388. KEYSERLINGK, H. (1950) 'Perritin.' [In German.] Psychiatrie,
      Neurologie, und Medizinische Psychologie, 2, 1-9.

389. KJELLBERG, B., and RANDRUP, A. (1973) 'Disruption of social
      behaviour of vervet monkeys (Cercopithecus) by low doses of
      amphetamines.' Pharmakopsychiatrie und Neuropsychopharma-
      kologie, 6, 287-293.

390. KLEDZIK, G.S., and MEITES, J. (1974) 'Reinitiation of estrous
      cycles in light-induced constant estrous female rats by
      drugs.' Proceedings of the Society for Experimental Biology
      and Medicine, 146, 989-992.

391. KNAPP, P.H. (1952) 'Amphetamine and addiction.' Journal of
      Nervous and Mental Diseases, 115, 406-432.

392. KRAMER, J.C., FISCHMAN, V.S., and LITTLEFIELD, D.C. (1967) 'Am-
      phetamine abuse: Pattern and effects of high doses taken
      intravenously.' Journal of the American Medical Association,
      201, 305-309.

393. LADEWIG, D., BATTEGAY, R., and LABHARDT, F. (1969) 'Stim-
      ulantien: Abhängigkeit und Psychosen.' ['Stimulants:
      Dependency and psychoses.'] Deutsche Medizinische Wochen-
      schrift, 94, 101-107.

394. LEWANDEN, T. (1977) 'Effects of amphetamine in animals.' In:
        W.R. Martin, ed. Drug Addiction II. New York: Springer-
        Verlag, pp. 3-246.

395. LIDZ, T., LIDZ, R., and RUBENSTEIN, R. (1976) 'An anaclitic
        syndrome in adolescent amphetamine addicts.' Psychoanalytic
        Study of the Child, 31, 317-348.

396. LINKEN, A. (1968) 'A study of drug-taking among young patients
        attending a clinic for venereal diseases.' British Journal
        of Venereal Diseases, 44, 337-341.

397. LOEWE, S. (1938) 'Ejaculation induced by drug action.' Ar-
        chives Internationales de Pharmacodynamie et de Therapie,
        60, 37-47.

398. MC CORMICK, T.C. (1962) 'Toxic reactions to the amphetamines.'
        Diseases of the Nervous System, 23, 219-223.

399. MEYERSON, B.J. (1968) 'Amphetamine and 5-hydroxytryptamine in-
        hibition of copulatory behaviour in the female rat.' Annales
        Mediciniae Experimentalis et Biologiae Fennicae, 46, 394-398.

400. MICHANEK, A. (1979) 'Potentiation of D- and L-amphetamine ef-
        fects on copulatory behavior in female rats by treatment with
        alpha-adrenoreceptor blocking drugs.' Archives Inter-
        nationales de Pharmacodynamie et de Therapie, 239, 241-256.

401. MICHANEK, A., and MEYERSON, B.J. (1975) 'Copulatory behavior in
        the female rat after amphetamine and amphetamine deriv-
        atives.' In: M. Sandler and C.L. Gessa, eds. Sexual Behav-
        ior: Pharmacology and Biochemistry. New York: Raven Press,
        pp. 51-57.

402. MICHANEK, A., and MEYERSON, B.J. (1977) 'A comparative study of
        different amphetamines on copulatory behavior and stereotype
        activity in the female rat.' Psychopharmacology, 53, 175-
        183.

403. MICHANEK, A., and MEYERSON, B.J. (1977) 'The effects of differ-
        ent amphetamines on copulatory behaviour and stereotypic
        activity in the female rat, after treatment with monoamine
        depletors and synthesis inhibitors.' Archives Inter-
        nationales de Pharmacodynamie et de Therapie, 229, 301-312.

404. MONROE, R.R., and DULL, H.J. (1947) 'Oral use of stimulants
        obtained from inhalers.' Journal of the American Medical
        Association, 135, 909-915.

405. MORPURGO, C., and THEOBALD, W. (1966) 'Behavioral reactions to
        amphetamine in reserpinized rats.' International Journal of
        Neuropharmacology, 5, 375-377.

406. MOTT, J., and RATHOD, N.H. (1976) 'Heroin misuse and delinquency
        in a new town.' British Journal of Psychiatry, 128, 428-435.

407. NAIL, R.L., GUNDERSON, E.K.K., and KOLB, D. (1974) 'Motives for drug use among light and heavy users.' Journal of Nervous and Mental Diseases, 159, 131-138.

408. NATIONAL INSTITUTE ON DRUG ABUSE. (1972) Use and Abuse of Amphetamine and Its Substitutes. Washington, D.C.: U.S. Government Printing Office.

409. NODA, H. (1950) 'Concerning wake-amine intoxication.' [In Japanese.] Kurume Igakkai Zasshi, 13, 294-298.

410. NORMAN, J., and SHEA, J.T. (1945) 'Acute hallucinases as a complication of addiction to amphetamine sulfate.' New England Journal of Medicine, 233, 270-271.

411. OFORI-AKYEAH, J., and LEWIS, R.A. (1972) 'Drug abuse among Ghanian medical students.' Ghana Medical Journal, 1, 383-387.

412. PETERSON, B.H., and SOMERVILLE, D.M. (1949) 'Excessive use of "benzedrine" by a psychopath.' Medical Journal of Australia, 2, 948-949.

413. PITTEL, S.M., and HOFER, R. (1972) 'The transition to amphetamine abuse.' In: E.H. Ellinwood and S. Cohen, eds. Current Concepts on Amphetamine Abuse. Washington, D.C.: U.S. Government Printing Office, pp. 169-176.

414. RADCLIFFE, B.E. (1974) 'MDA.' Clinical Toxicology, 7, 405-411.

415. REED, D., CRANY, R., and SEDGWICK, A. (1972) 'A fetal case involving methylenedioxyamphetamine.' Clinical Toxicology, 5, 3-6.

416. RILEY, D.N., JAMIESON, B.D., and RUSSELL, P.N. (1971) 'A survey of drug use at the University of Canterbury.' New Zealand Medical Journal, 74, 365-368.

417. RIS, F. (1952) 'Bericht über langjahrigen Gebrauch mit Perritin in steigenden Dosen.' ['Report of year-long use of Perritin in increasing doses.'] Münchener Medizinische Wochenschrift, 94, 1039.

418. ROBINS, L.N., DARVISH, H.S., and MURPHY, G.E. (1970) 'The long-term outcome for adolescent drug users: A follow-up study of 76 users and 146 nonusers.' Proceedings of the American Psychopathological Association, 59, 159-180.

419. ROCKWELL, D.A., and OSTWALD, P. (1968) 'Amphetamine use and abuse in psychiatric patients.' Archives of General Psychiatry, 18, 612-616.

420. ROWAN, R.L., and HOWLEY, T.F. (1965) 'Ejaculatory sterility.' Fertility and Sterility, 16, 768.

421. ROX, W. (1959) 'Arzneimittelsucht durch Missbrauch von sogenann-
      ten Appetitzuglern.' ['Drug addiction by abuse of the so-
      called appetite depressants.'] Archiv für Toxikologie, 17,
      331-335.

422. RYLANDER, G. (1969) 'Clinical and medico-criminological aspects
      of addiction to central stimulating drugs.' In: F. Sjo-
      qvist and M. ToHie, eds. Abuse of Central Stimulants.
      New York: Raven Press, pp. 251-273.

423. SCHILDEN, P. (1938) 'The psychological effect of benzedrine
      sulfate.' Journal of Nervous and Mental Diseases, 87, 584.

424. SCHIORRING, E. (1977) 'Changes in individual and social behav-
      ior induced by amphetamine and related compounds in monkeys
      and man.' In: E.H. Ellinwood and M. Kilbey, eds. Cocaine
      and Other Stimulants. New York: Plenum Press, pp. 481-522.

425. SCOTT, P.D., and WILCOX, D.R.C. (1965) 'Delinquency and the
      amphetamines.' British Journal of Psychiatry, 111, 865-875.

426. SHICK, J.F., SMITH, D.E., and WESSON, D.R. (1972) 'An analysis
      of amphetamine toxicity and patterns of use.' Journal of
      Psychedelic Drugs, 5, 113-130.

427. SMITH, D.E., WESSON, D.R., BUXTON, M.E., SEYMOUR, R.B., UNGER-
      LEIDER, J.T., MORGAN, J.P., MANDELL, A.J., and JARA, G.
      (1979) 'Amphetamine abuse and sexual dysfunctions:
      Clinical and research considerations.' In: D.E. Smith,
      ed. Amphetamine Use, Misuse, and Abuse. Cambridge:
      G.K. Hall, pp. 228-265.

428. SMITH, D.E., and LUCE, J. (1971) Love Needs Care. Boston,
      Massachusetts: Little, Brown, and Company.

429. SOULAIRAC, M.-L. (1963) 'Étude expérimentale des regulations
      hormonerveuses du comportement sexuel du rat male.' ['Exper-
      imental study of the regulation of hormonal nerves in the
      sexual behavior of the male rat.'] Annales de Endocrin-
      ologie, 24 (Supplement), 1-98.

430. SOULAIRAC, M.-L., and SOULAIRAC, A. (1972) 'Action des sub-
      stances neurostimulantes sur le comportement sexuel du rat
      male apres lesions du cortex cerebral.' ['Action of neuro-
      stimulating substances on the sexual behavior of the male
      rat after lesions of the cerebral cortex.'] Journal de
      Physiologie, 65, 504A (abstract).

431. STAEHELIN, J.E. (1941) 'Perritin-Psychose.' ['Perritin psy-
      chosis.'] Zeitschrift für die Gesamte Neurologie und Psy-
      chiatrie, 173, 598-620.

432. STOFFER, S.S., SAPIRA, J.D., TWEEDDALE, D.N., and MEKETON, B.F.
      (1969) 'Effect of D-amphetamine on menstruation.' American
      Journal of Obstetrics and Gynecology, 105, 989-990.

433. TOPORSKAIA, N.A. (1975) 'Effect of certain neurotropic drugs
     on the process of ovulation.' [In Russian.] Akusherstvo
     Ginekologiia, 10, 13-15.

434. TRIMBLE, G.X. (1960) 'Drug-induced impotence?' Journal of the
     American Medical Association, 174, 2095.

435. TUREK, I.S., SOSKIN, R.A., and KURLAND, A.A. (1974) 'Methylene-
     dioxyamphetamine (MDA): Subjective effects.' Journal of
     Psychedelic Drugs, 6, 7-14.

436. WAND, S.P. (1938) 'Effects of toxic doses of benzyl methylcar-
     binamine (Benzedrine) in man.' Journal of the American
     Medical Association, 110, 206-207.

437. WEIL, A. (1976) 'The love drug.' Journal of Psychedelic Drugs,
     8, 335-337.

438. WIECKMAN, F.H. (1960) 'Drug-induced impotence.' Journal of the
     American Medical Association, 174, 2096.

439. ZEMLAN, F.P., TRULSON, M.E., HOWELL, R., and HOEBEL, B.G. (1977)
     'Influence of P-chloroamphetamine on female sexual reflexes
     and brain monoamine levels.' Brain Research, 123, 347-356.

440. ZINBERG, N.E. (1976) 'Observations on the phenomenology of con-
     sciousness change.' Journal of Psychedelic Drugs, 8, 59-76.

441. ZONDEK, L. (1958) 'Amphetamine abuse and its relation to other
     drug addictions.' Psychiatria et Neurologia, 135, 227-246.

Antidepressants

442. BAI, J., GREENWALD, E., CATERINI, H., and KAMINETZKY, H. (1974) 'Drug-related menstrual aberrations.' Obstetrics and Gynecology, 44, 713-719

443. BARTON, J. L. (1979) 'Orgasmic inhibition by phenelzine.' American Journal of Psychiatry, 136, 1616-1617

444. BEAUMONT, G. (1977) 'Sexual side-effects of clomipramine (Anafranil).' Journal of International Medical Research, 5 (Supplement), 37-44.

445. BENKERT, O. (1980) 'Pharmacotherapy of sexual impotence in the male.' Modern Problems in Pharmacopsychiatry, 15, 158-173.

446. BENNETT, D. (1961) 'Treatment of ejaculatio praecox with monoamine oxidase inhibitors.' Lancet, 2, 1309.

447. BODNAR, S., and CATTERILL, T. B. (1972) 'Amitriptyline in emotional states associated with the climacteric.' Psychosomatics, 13, 117-119.

448. BUTCHER, L. L., BUTCHER, S. G., AND LARSSON, K. (1969) 'Effects of apomorphine (+)-amphetamine, and nialamide on tetrabenazine-induced suppression of sexual behavior in the male rat. European Journal of Pharmacology, 7, 283-288.

449. CLARKE, F. C. (1969). 'The treatment of depression in general practice.' South African Medical Journal, 43, 724-725.

450. COMFORT, A. (1979) 'Effects of psychoactive drugs on ejaculation.' American Journal of Psychiatry, 136, 124-125.

451. COUPER-SMARTT, J. D., and RCDHAM, R. (1973) 'A technique for
          surveying side effects of tricyclic drugs with reference
          to reported sexual effects.' Journal of International
          Medical Research, 1, 473-476.

452. DAVIS, J., CLYMAN, M. J., DECKER, A., BRONSTEIN, S., and ROLAND,
          M. (1966). 'Effect of phenelzine on semin in infertility:
          A preliminary report. Fertility and Sterility, 17,
          221-224.

453. DEWSBURY, D. A. (1975) 'The normal heterosexual pattern of
          copulatory behavior in male rats: Effects of drugs that
          alter brain monoamine levels.' In Sandler, M. and Gessa,
          G. L. (editors). Sexual Behavior: Pharmacology and
          Biochemistry. New York: Raven Press, 169-179.

454. DEWSBURY, D. A., DAVIS, H. N., and JANSEN, P. E. (1972) 'Effects
          of monoamine oxidase inhibitors on the copulatory
          behavior of male rats. Psychopharmacology, 24, 209-217.

455. ELLINWOOD, E. H., and ROCKWELL, K. (1975) 'The effect of
          drug use on sexual behavior.' Medical Aspects of
          Human Sexuality, 9, 10-12.

456. EVERETT, H. C. (1975) 'The use of bethanechol chloride with
          tricyclic antidepressants. American Journal of
          Psychiatry, 132, 1202-1204.

457. GAWIN, F. H. (1978) 'Drugs and eros: Reflection on aphrodisiacs.'
          Journal of Psychedelic Drugs, 10, 227-236.

458. GESSA, G. L., and TAGLIAMONTE, A. (1973) 'Role of brain
          monoamines in controlling sexual behavior in male animals.'
          In Ban, T. A., Boissier, J. R., Gessa, G. J., Heinmann, L,
          and Hollister, L. (editors). Psychopharmacology,
          Sexual Disorders And Drug Abuse. Amsterdam: North-Holland
          Publishing Co., 451-462.

459. GESSA, G. L., and TAGLIAMONTE, A. (1975) 'Role of brain
          serotonin and dopamine in male sexual behavior.' In
          Sandler, M. and Gessa, G. L. (editors). Sexual Behavior:
          Pharmacology and Biochemistry. New York: Raven Press,
          117-128.

460. GIRGIS, S., ETRIBY, A., EL-HEFNAWY, H., and KAHIL, S. (1968)
          'Aspermia: A survey of 40 cases.' Fertility and Sterility,
          19, 580-588.

461. GLASS, R. (1981) 'Ejaculatory impairment from both phenelzine
          and imipramine with tinnitus from phenelzine.' Journal
          of Clinical Psychopharmacology, 1, 152-154.

462. GREENBERG, H. R. (1965) 'Erectile impotence during the course of
          Tofranil therapy.' American Journal of Psychiatry,
          121, 1021.

463. GWIN, R. D. and O'HARA, G. L. (1978) 'Drug induced changes
         in sexuality.' Apothecary, January, 11-60.

464. HEKIMIAN, L., FRIEDHOFF, A., and DEEVER, E. 91978) 'A com-
         parison of the onset of action and therapeutic efficacy
         of amoxapine and amitriptyline.' Journal of Clinical
         Psychiatry, 39, 633-637.

465. HOLLINFIELD, J. W., SHERMAN, K., VANDER ZWAGG, R., and SHAND, D.
         (1976) 'Proposed mechanisms of propranolol's anti-
         hypertensive effect in essential hypertension.' New
         England Journal of Medicine, 295, 68-73.

466. HORWITZ, D., and SJOERDSMA, A. (1961) 'A non'hydrazine mono-
         amine oxidase inhibitor with antihypertensive properties.'
         Proceedings of the Society for Experimental Biology and
         Medicine, 106, 118-120.

467. KEDIA, K., and MARKLAND, C. (1975) 'The effect of pharmaco-
         logical agents on ejaculation.' Journal of Urology,
         114, 569-573.

468. KERR, M. M. (1970) 'Amitriptyline in emotional states at the
         menopause.' New Zealand Medical Journal, 72, 243-245.

469. KOHN, R. M. (1964) 'Nocturnal orthostatic syncope in pargyline
         therapy.' Journal of the American Medical Association,
         187, 229-230.

470. KULIK, F., and WILBUR, R. (1982) 'Case report of painful
         ejaculation as a side effect of amoxapine.' American
         Journal of Psychiatry, 139, 234-235.

471. KURLAND, A. A., PINTO, A., DESTOUNIS, N., and BABIKOW, P. W.
         (1970) 'Effects of trimipramine (Surmontil) on sperm-
         atogenesis and mood in normal volunteers.' Current
         Therapy and Research, 12, 186-190.

472. LEVIN, R. M., AMSTERDAM, J. D., WINOKUR, A., and WEIN, A. J.
         (1981) 'Effects of psychotropic drugs on human sperm
         motility.' Fertility and Sterility, 36, 503-506.

473. LEVIN, R. M., SHOTEN, J., GREENBERG, S. H. (1980) A
         quantitative method for determining the effects of drugs
         on spermatozoal motility.' Fertility and Sterility,
         33, 631-634.

474. LOVECKY, D. V., and DEWSBURY, D. A. (1973) 'Effects of
         imipramine on copulatory behavior of male rats.'
         Bulletin of the Psychonomic Society, 2, 237-239.

475. MYERSON, B. J. (1964) 'Central nervous monoamines and hormone-
         induced estrous behaviour in the spayed rat.' Acta
         Physiologica Scandinavica, 53 (Supplement), 241.

476. MYERSON, B. J. (1964) 'The effect of neuropharmacological agents

on hormone-activated estrous behaviour in ovariectomized rats. Archives International de Pharmacodynamie et de Therapie, 150, 4-]0.

477. MYERSON, B. J. (1966) 'Oestrous behavior in oestrogen treated ovariectomized rats after chlorpromazine alone or in combination with progesterone, tetrabenazine or reserpine.' Acta Pharmacologica et Toxicologica, 24, 363-369.

478. MYERSON, B. J. (1975) 'Drugs and sexual motivation in the female rat.' In Sandler, M. and Gessa, G. L. (editors). Sexual Behavior: Pharmacology and Biochemistry. New York: Raven Press, 21-31.

479. NININGER, J. E.   (1978) 'Inhibition of ejaculation by amitriptyline.' American Journal of Psychiatry, 135, 750-751.

480. PETRIE, W. M. (1980) 'Sexual effects of antidepressants and psychomotor stimulant drugs.' Modern Problems in Pharmacopsychiatry, 15, 77-90.

481. RAPP, M. (1979) 'Two cases of ejaculatory impairment related to phenelzine.' American Journal of Psychiatry, 136, 1200-1201.

482. RUSKIN, D. B., and GOLDNER, R. D. (1959) 'Treatment of depressions in private practice with imimpramine.' Diseases of the Nervous System, 20, 391-399.

483. SCHWARTZ, N. H., and ROBINSON, B. D. (1952) 'Impotence due to methantheline bromide.' New York State Journal of Medicine, 52, 1530.

484. SIMPSON, G. M., BLAIR, J. H., and AMUSO, D. (1965) 'Effects of antidepressants on genito-urinary function.' Diseases of the Nervous System, 26, 787-789.

485. URRY, R. L., DOUGHERTY, K. A., and COCKETT, A. T. K. (1976) 'Age-related changes in male rat reproductive organ weights and plasma testosterone concentrations after administration of a monoamine oxidase inhibitor.' Fertility and Sterility, 27, 1326-1334.

486. WYATT, R. J., FRAM, D., BUCHBINDER, R., and SNYDER, F. (1971) 'Treatment of intractable narcolepsy with a monoamine oxidase inhibitor.' New England Journal of Medicine, 285, 987-991.

Antipsychotics

487.   AMDUR, M.   (1976)   'Confirming a side effect.'   American
       Journal of Psychiatry, 133, 864-865.

488.   BARRACLOUGH, C., and SAWYER, C.   (1957)   'Blockage of the
       release of pituitary ovulating hormone in the rat by
       chlorpromazine and reserpine: Possible mechanisms of
       action.'   Endocrinology, 61, 341-351.

489.   BARRACLOUGH, C.A., and SAWYER, C.   (1959)   'Induction of
       pseudopregnancy in the rat by reserpine and chlorpro-
       mazine.'   Endocrinology, 65, 563-571.

490.   BARTHOLOMEW, A.A.   (1968)   'A long-acting phenothiazine
       as a possible agent to control deviant sexual behaviour.'
       American Journal of Psychiatry, 124, 917-923.

491.   BENKERT, O.   (1980)   'Pharmacotherapy of sexual impotence
       in the male.'   Modern Problems of Pharmacopsychology,
       15, 158-173.

492.   BERGER, S.H.   (1979)   'Trifluoperazine and haloperidal:
       Sources of ejaculatory pain?'   American Journal of
       Psychiatry, 136, 350.

493.   BHARGAVA, K.P., and JAITLY, K.D.   (1964)   'The effect of some
       phenothiazine tranquilizers on the oestrous cycle of
       albino mice.'   British Journal of Pharmacology, 22,
       162-165.

494.   BLAIR, J.H., and SIMPSON, G.M.   (1966)   'Effect of anti-
       psychotic drugs on reproductive functions.'   Diseases
       of the Nervous System, 27, 645-647.

495.   BROWN, W.A., LAUGHREN, T., and WILLIAMS, B.   (1981)   'Dif-
       ferential effects of neuroleptic agents on the pituitary-
       gonadal axis in men.'   Archives of General Psychiatry,
       38, 1270-1272.

496. BYCK, R. (1975) 'Drugs and the treatment of psychiatric dis-
     orders.' In: L. Goodman and A. Gilman, eds. The Pharm-
     acological Basis of Therapeutics. New York: Macmillan
     Publishing Company.

497. CLARK, M.L., and JOHNSON, P.C. (1960) 'Amenorrhea and elevated
     levels of serum cholesterol produced by trifluoromethylated
     phenothiazine.' Journal of Clinical Endocrinology, 20,
     641-646.

498. CLEIN, L. (1962) 'Thioridazine and ejaculation.' British
     Medical Journal, 2, 548-549.

499. COHEN, I. (1956) 'Complications of chlorpromazine therapy.'
     American Journal of Psychiatry, 113, 115-121.

500. CORTEZ, P.E., and DURAZO, Q.F. (1963) 'Alteraciones endocrinas
     observadas en pacientés bajo tratamiento con trifluopera-
     zine.' ['Endocrine alterations observed in patients treated
     with trifluoperazine.'] Revista de Medicina de Hospital
     General, 26, 883-888.

501. DATSHKOVSKY, J. (1961) 'Mellaril: Ejaculation disorders.'
     American Journal of Psychiatry, 118, 564.

502. DITMAN, K.S. (1964) 'Inhibition of ejaculation by chlorpro-
     thixene.' American Journal of Psychiatry, 120, 1004-1005.

503. DORMAN, B.W., and SCHMIDT, J.D. (1976) 'Association of priapism
     in phenothiazine therapy.' Journal of Urology, 116, 5153.

504. DOTTI, A., and REDA, M. (1975) 'Major tranquilizers and sexual
     function.' In: M. Sandler and G.L. Gessa, eds. Sexual
     Behavior: Pharmacology and Biochemistry. New York: Raven
     Press, pp. 193-195.

505. FOOTE, R.H., and GRAY, L.C. (1960) 'Effect of promazine hydro-
     chloride and chlorpromazine hydrochloride on the motility
     and fertility of bovine semen.' Journal of Dairy Science,
     43, 1499-1504.

506. FOOTE, R.H., and GARY, L.C. (1963) 'Effect of tranquilizers
     on libido, sperm production and in vitro sperm survival in
     dogs.' Proceedings of the Society for Experimental Bio-
     logy and Medicine, 114, 396-398.

507. FREYHAN, F.A. (1961) 'Loss of ejaculation during Mellaril
     treatment.' American Journal of Psychiatry, 118, 171-172.

508. GILLETTE, E. (1960) 'Effects of chlorpromazine and d-lysergic
     acid diethylamide on sex behavior of male rats.' Pro-
     ceedings of the Society for Experimental Biology and
     Medicine, 103, 392-394.

509. GIRGIS, S., ETRIBY, A., EL-HEFNAWY, H., and KAHIL, S. (1968) 'Aspermia: A survey of 40 cases.' Fertility and Sterility, 19, 580-588.

510. GREEN, M. (1961) 'Inhibition of ejaculation as a side-effect of mellaril.' American Journal of Psychiatry, 118, 172-173.

511. GREENBERG, H.R. (1971) 'Inhibition of ejaculation by chlorpromazine.' Journal of Nervous and Mental Disease, 152, 364-366.

512. GREENBERG, H.R., and CARRILLO, C. (1968) 'Thioridazine-induced inhibition of masturbatory ejaculation in an adolescent.' American Journal of Psychiatry, 124, 991-993.

513. HAFS, H.D., and WILLIAMS, J.A. (1964) 'The effects of prolonged chlorpromzaine administration on the reproductive organs in the rat.' American Journal of Veterinary Research, 25, 523-527.

514. HAIDER, I. (1966) 'Thioridazine and sexual dysfunctions.' International Journal of Neuropsychiatry, 2, 255-257.

515. HEILER, J. (1961) 'Another case of inhibition of ejaculation as a side effect of mellaril.' American Journal of Psychiatry, 118, 173.

516. HOLLISTER, L.E. (1964) 'Adverse reactions to phenothiazines.' Journal of the American Medical Association, 189, 311-313.

517. HOLLISTER, L.E. (1964) 'Complications from psychotherapeutic drugs.' Clinical Pharmacology and Therapeutics, 5, 322-333.

518. JARRETT, R.J. (1963) 'Some endocrine effects of two phenothiazine derivatives, chlorpromazine and perphenazine, in the female mouse.' British Journal of Pharmacology, 20, 497-506.

519. KOTIN, J., WILBERT, D.E., VERBURG, D., and SOLDINGER, S.M. (1976) 'Thioridazine and sexual dysfunction.' American Journal of Psychiatry, 133, 82-85.

520. LAUGHREN, T.P., BROWN, W., and PETRUCCI, J. (1978) 'Effects of thioridazine on serum testosterone.' American Journal of Psychiatry, 135, 982-984.

521. MONEY, J., and YANKOWITZ, R. (1967) 'The sympathetic-inhibiting effects of the drug ismelin on human male eroticism with a note on mellaril.' Journal of Sex Research, 3, 69-82.

522. NIMH COLLABORATIVE STUDY GROUP. (1964) 'Phenothiazine treatment in acute schizophrenia.' Archives of General Psychiatry, 10, 246-261.

523. POLISHUK, W.Z., and FLIGELMAN, S. (1956) 'Chlorpromazine and amenorrhea.' Lancet, 2, 465-466.

524. POLISHUK, W.Z., and KULCSAR, S. (1956) 'Effects of chlorpromazine on pituitary function.' Journal of Clinical Endocrinology, 16, 292-293.

525. PSYCHOYOS, A. (1968) 'The effects of reserpine and chlorpromazine on sexual function.' Journal of Reproduction and Fertility, Supplement 4, 47-60.

526. RUBIN, R.T., POLAND, R.E., and TOWER, B.B. (1976) 'Prolactin-related testosterone secretion in normal adult men.' Journal of Clinical Endocrinology and Metabolism, 42, 112-116.

527. SANDISON, R.A., WHITELAW, E., and CURRIE, J.D.C. (1960) 'Clinical trials with melleril in the treatment of schizophrenia.' Journal of Mental Science, 106, 732-741.

528. SHADER, R.I. (1964) 'Sexual dysfunction associated with thioridazine hydrochloride.' Journal of the American Medical Association, 188, 1007-1009.

529. SHADER, R.I. (1970) 'Endocrine, metabolic, and genitourinary effects of psychotropic drugs.' In: A. DiMascia and R.I. Shader, eds. Clinical Handbook of Psychopharmacology. New York: Science House, pp. 205-212.

530. SHADER, R.I. (1972) 'Sexual dysfunction associated with mesoridazine besylate (Serentil).' Psychopharmacologia, 27, 293-294.

531. SHADER, R.I., and DI MASCIA, A. (1970) Psychotropic Drug Side Effects. Baltimore, Md.: Williams and Wilkins Co.

532. SHADER, R.I., and GRINSPOON, L. (1967) 'Schizophrenia, oligospermia, and the phenothiazines.' Diseases of the Nervous System, 28, 240-244.

533. SHADER, R.I., TAYMOR, M.L., and GRINSPOON, L. (1968) 'Schizophrenia, oligospermia, and the phenothiazines. II. Studies on follicle stimulating hormone.' Proceedings IV World Congress of Psychiatry. Excerpta Medica International Congress Series, 150, 640-643.

534. SHIBUSAWA, K., SAITO, S., FUKUDA, M., KAWAI, T., YAMADA, H., and TOMIZAWA, K. (1955) 'Inhibition of the hypothalamo-neurohypophyseal neurosecretion by chlorpromazine.' Endocrinologia Japonica, 2 189-194.

535.   SINGH, H. (1961) 'A case of inhibition of ejaculation
           as a side effect of Mellaril.' American Journal of
           Psychiatry, 117, 1041-1042.

536.   STORY, N.L. (1974) 'Sexual dysfunction resulting from
           drug side effects.' Journal of Sex Research, 10,
           132-149.

537.   SULMAN, F.G., and WINNIK, H.S. (1956) 'Hormonal effects of
           chlorpromazine.' Lancet, 1, 161-162.

538.   TAUBEL, D. (1961) 'Mellaril: Ejaculation disorders.'
           American Journal of Psychiatry, 119, 87.

539.   TENNENT, G., BANCROFT, J., and CASS, J. (1974) 'The control
           of devient sexual behavior by drugs: A doubleblind
           controlled study of benperidol, chlorpromazine, and
           placebo.' Archives of Sexual Behavior, 3, 261-271.

540.   WALLACH, E.E., GARCIA, C., and PINCUS, G. (1965) 'Anovulation
           in hospitalized mental patients.' American Journal of
           Obstetrics and Gynecology, 93, 72-78.

541.   WELLS, H., BRIGGS, F.N., and MUNSON, P.L. (1956) 'The
           inhibitor effect of reserpine on ACTH secretion in
           response to stressful stimuli.' Endocrinology, 59,
           571-579.

542.   WHITELAW, M.L. (1956) 'Delay in ovulation and menstruation
           induced by chlorpromazine.' Journal of Clinical Endo-
           crinology, 16, 972.

543.   WITTON, K. (1962) 'Sexual dysfunction secondary to Mellaril.'
           Diseases of the Nervous System, 23, 175.

Barbiturates

544. ADAMS, T.E., and SPIES, H.G. (1981) 'GnRH-induced regulation of GnRH receptor concentration in the phenobarbital-blocked hamster.' Biology of Reproduction, 25, 298-302.

545. AHMED, S.H. (1968) 'Treatment of premature ejaculation.' British Journal of Psychiatry, 114, 1197-1198.

546. ASHIRU, O.A., and BLAKE, C.A. (1979) 'Stimulation of endogenous follicle-stimulating hormone release during estrus by exogenous follicle-stimulating hormone or luteinizing hormone at proestrus in the phenobarbital-blocked rat.' Endocrinology, 105, 1162-1167.

547. BACKSTROM, T., and JORPES, P. (1979) 'Serum phenytoin, phenobarbital, carbamazepine, albumin; and plasma estradiol, progesterone concentrations during the menstrual cycle in women with epilepsy.' Acta Neurologica Scandinavica, 59, 63-71.

548. BARR, G.D., and BARRACLOUGH, C.A. (1978) 'Temporal changes in medial basal hypothalamic LH-RH correlated with plasma LH during the rat estrus cycle and following electrochemical stimulation of the medial preoptic area in pentobarbital-treated proestrous rats.' Brain Research, 148, 413-423.

549. BEATTIE, C.W., CAMPBELL, C.S., NEQUIN, L.G., SOYHA, L.F., and SCHWARTZ, N.B. (1973) 'Barbiturate blockade of tonic LH secretion in the male and female rat.' Endocrinology, 92, 1630-1638.

550. BLAKE, C.A. (1976) 'Simulation of the early phase of the proestrous follicle-stimulating hormone rise after infusion of luteinizing hormone-releasing hormone in phenobarbital-blocked rats.' Endocrinology, 98, 461-467.

551.   BLAKE, C.A.   (1976)   'Simulation of the proestrous luteinizing
       hormone (LH) surge after infusion of LH-releasing hormone
       in phenobarbital-blocked rats.'   Endocrinology, 98, 451-460.

552.   BROWN-GRANT, K.   (1969)   'The effects of progesterone and of
       pentobarbitone administered at the dioestrous stage on the
       ovarian cycle of the rat.'   Journal of Endocrinology, 43,
       539-552.

553.   CHAPPEL, S.C., and BARRACLOUGH, C.A.   (1976)   'The effects of
       sodium pentobarbital or ether anesthesia on spontaneous and
       electrochemically-induced gonadotropin release.'   Pro-
       ceedings of the Society for Experimental Biology and
       Medicine, 153, 1-6.

554.   CHATEAU, D., and ARON, C.   (1973)   'Demonstration of an effect of
       pentobarbital on the length of the estrus cycle in the
       female rat.'   [In French.]   Comptes Rendus des Seances de la
       Société de Biologie, 167, 366-368.

555.   COUTIFARIS, C., and CHAPPEL, S.C.   (1982)   'Intraventricular
       injection of follicle-stimulating hormone (FSH) during pro-
       estrus stimulates the rise in serum FSH on estrus in pento-
       barbital-treated hamsters through a central nervous system-
       dependent mechanism.'   Endocrinology, 110, 105-113.

556.   DAMBER, J.E., CARSTENSEN, H., and LINDGREN, S.   (1977)   'The
       effects of barbiturate anesthesia and laparotomy in testis
       and plasma testosterone in rats.'   Journal of Steroid Bio-
       chemistry, 8, 217-219.

557.   DOMINGUEZ, R., and SMITH, E.R.   (1974)   'Barbiturate blockade of
       ovulation on days other than proestrus in the rat.'   Neuro-
       endocrinology, 14, 212-223.

558.   DYER, R.G., and MANSFIELD, S.   (1980)   'Relationship between
       duration of urethane or pentobarbitone anaesthesia in male
       and female rats and adenohypophyseal response to luteinizing
       hormone-releasing hormone.'   British Journal of Pharmacology,
       69, 139-143.

559.   DYER, R.G., and MAYES, L.C.   (1978)   'Electrical stimulation of
       the hypothalamus: New observations on the parameters
       necessary for ovulation in rats anaesthetised with pento-
       barbitone during the pro-oestrous "critical period."'
       Experimental Brain Research, 33, 583-592.

560.   EVERETT, J.W.   (1967)   'Provoked ovulation or long-delayed
       pseudo-pregnancy from coital stimuli in barbiturate-
       blocked rats.'   Endocrinology, 80, 145-154.

561.   FAHIM, M.S., KING, T.M., VENSON, V., NORWICH, C., and BOLT, D.J.
        (1969) 'Uterotropic action of estrogens in phenobarbital-
        treated mice.' Fertility and Sterility, 20, 344-350.

562.   FURUDATE, S. (1975) 'On the activation of the corpus luteum of
        the rat estrous cycle with phenobarbital anesthesia. I. In-
        duction of pseudopregnancy by a single subcutaneous injec-
        tion of phenobarbital.' Kitasato Archives of Experimental
        Medicine, 48, 131-139.

563.   FURUDATE, S. (1977) 'On the activation of the corpus luteum of
        rat estrous cycle with phenobarbital anesthesia. II. Block-
        ade by luteinizing hormone of phenobarbital-induced pseudo-
        pregnancy.' Kitasato Archives of Experimental Medicine, 50,
        47-56.

564.   HAGINO, N. (1979) 'Effect of nembutal on LH release in baboons.'
        Hormone and Metabolic Research, 11, 296-300.

565.   HAGINO, N., RAMALEY, J.A., and GORSKI, R.A. (1966) 'Inhibition
        of estrogen-induced precocious ovulation by pentobarbital
        in the rat.' Endocrinology, 79, 451-454.

566.   HASEGAWA, Y., MIYAMOTO, K., YAZAKI, C., and IGARASHI, M. (1981)
        'Regulation of the second surge of follicle-stimulating
        hormone: Effects of antiluteinizing hormone-releasing
        hormone serum and pentobarbital.' Endocrinology, 109, 130-
        135.

567.   KALRA, S.P., SIMPKINS, J.W., and KALRA, P.S. (1981) 'Pro-
        gesterone-induced changes in hypothalamic luteinizing hor-
        mone-releasing hormone and catecholamines: Differential
        effects of pentobarbital.' Endocrinology, 108, 1299-1304.

568.   KANEKO, S. (1980) 'Changes in plasma progestin, prolactin, LH,
        and FH at luteal activation with phenobarbital anesthesia
        in the rat.' Endocrinology, 27, 431-438.

569.   KIMURA, F., KAWAKAMI, M., NAKANO, H., and MC CANN, S.M. (1980)
        'Changes in adenosine 3',5'-monophosphate and guanosine
        3',5'-monophosphate concentrations in the anterior pituitary
        and hypothalamus during the rat estrous cycle and effects
        of administration of sodium pentobarbital in proestrus.'
        Endocrinology, 106, 631-635.

570.   KOBAYASHI, F., HARA, K., and MIYAKE, T. (1973) 'Facilitation by
        progesterone of ovulating hormone release in sodium pento-
        barbital-blocked proestrous rats.' Endocrinology, 20, 175-
        180.

571.   KRAFT, T. (1968) 'Treatment of premature ejaculation.' British
        Journal of Psychiatry, 114, 1595-1596.

572. LEONARDI, R., and CIACCIO, C. (1967) 'Observations on the
       morphofunctional changes induced by a barbiturate (pentothal)
       on the genitals of female rats.' Rivista Ostetrica-Gineco-
       logia, 22, 351-360.

573. LEVIN, W., WELCH, R.M., and CONNEY, A.H. (1969) 'Inhibitory
       effect of phenobarbital or chlordane pretreatment on the
       androgen-induced increase in seminal vescicle weight in the
       rat.' Steroids, 13, 155-161.

574. MANSAT, H.K. (1980) 'Effects of few anesthetics on testosterone
       concentration in testis and plasma of the rhesus monkey
       Macaca mulatta.' Indian Journal of Experimental Biology,
       18, 405-406.

575. MC CORMACK, C.E., and MANN, B.G. (1974) 'Reversal by proges-
       terone of barbiturate blockade of ovulation: Effect on
       concentration of serum LH.' Proceedings of the Society
       for Experimental Biology and Medicine, 146, 329-332.

576. MC CORMACK, C.E., and STRAUSS, W.F. (1975) 'Reversal by pro-
       gesterone of phenobarbitone-blockade by ovulation in the
       prepubertal rat primed with pregnant mare serum gonado-
       tropin.' Journal of Endocrinology, 65, 177-182.

577. MEYER, M.H., MASKEN, J.F., NETT, T.M., and NISWANDER, G.D.
       (1974) 'Serum levels of gonadotropin-releasing hormone
       (GN-RH) during the estrous cycle and in pentobarbital-
       treated rats.' Neuroendocrinology, 15, 32-37.

578. MEYER, R.R., KARAVOLAS, H.J., KLAUSING, M., and NORGARD, P.W.
       (1971) 'Blood progesterone and pregnenolone levels during
       phenobarbital (PB) block of PMS-induced ovulation in im-
       mature rats.' Endocrinology, 88, 983-990.

579. NAIL, R.L., GUNDERSON, E.F., and KOLB, D. (1974) 'Motives for
       drug use among light and heavy users.' Journal of Nervous
       and Mental Diseases, 159, 131-136.

580. NAKAMURA, Y., and UEDA, S. (1980) 'Induction of testosterone
       16 betahydroxylase in rat liver microsomes by phenobarbital
       pretreatment.' Biochemical and Biophysical Research Com-
       munications, 93, 1014-1019.

581. NAKAMURA, Y., and UEDA, S. (1980) 'Sixteen beta-hydroxylation
       of 4-androstene-3,17-dione in phenobarbital-pretreated rat
       liver microsomes.' FEBS Letters, 113, 193-195.

582. NORMAN, R.L., BLAKE, C.A., and SAWYER, C.H. (1972) 'Delay of
       the proestrous ovulatory surge of LH in the hamster by
       pentobarbital or ether.' Endocrinology, 91, 1025-1029.

583. NORMAN, R.L., BLAKE, C.A., and SAWYER, C.H. (1973) 'Evidence for
      neural sites of action of phenobarbital and progesterone on
      LH release in the hamster.' Biology of Reproduction, 8,
      83-86.

584. NORMAN, R.L., and GREENWALD, G.S. (1971) 'Effect of phenobar-
      bital, hypophysectomy, and x-irradiation on preovulatory
      progesterone levels in the cyclic hamster.' Endocrinology,
      89, 598-605.

585. OSMAN, P., and MEIJS-ROELOFS, H.F. (1976) 'Effects of sodium
      pentobarbitone administration on gonadotrophin release,
      first ovulation and ovarian morphology in pubertal rats.'
      Journal of Endocrinology, 68, 431-437.

586. OYAMA, C., MAEDA, T., and KUDO, T. (1973) 'Effects of thio-
      pental nitrous-oxide anesthesia and surgical stress on
      concentration of testosterone in human blood.' [In Japan-
      ese.] Horumon To Rinsho [Clinical Endocrinology], 21, 537-
      539.

587. PANCHENKO, E.N. (1969) 'On the treatment of ejaculatio praecox.'
      [In Russian.] Sovetskaia Meditsina, 32, 134-136.

588. PANDEY, S.D., and DOMINIC, C.J. (1980) 'Effect of nembutal
      anaesthesia on male induction of estrus (the Whitten ef-
      fect) in the wild mouse Mus musculus domesticus.' Indian
      Journal of Experimental Biology, 18, 445-446.

589. PAUP, D.C. (1973) 'Effect of progesterone and nembutal in
      altering estrous running and vaginal periodicity in the
      female rat.' Endocrinology, 92, 1530-1535.

590. PRESL, J. (1975) 'Modification of the biological activity of
      estrogens by means of barbiturates and induction of ovu-
      lation.' [In Czech.] Ceskoslovenska Gynekologie, 40,
      756-757.

591. PROP-VAN DEN BERG, C.M., SCHUURMAN, T., and WIEPKEMA, P.R. (1977)
      'Nembutal treatment of the VMH (rat): Effects on feeding
      and sexual behavior.' Brain Research, 126, 519-529.

592. RANCE, N., and BARRACLOUGH, C.A. (1981) 'Effects of pheno-
      barbital on hypothalamic LHRH and catecholamine turnover
      rates in proestrous rats.' Proceedings of the Society for
      Experimental Biology and Medicine, 166, 425-431.

593. ROZANOVA, V.D. (1979) 'Relationship between the phase of the
      sex cycle and differences in the rate of hexenal detox-
      ication and its induction by phenobarbital in female rats.'
      [In Russian.] Farmakologiia i Toksikologiia, 42, 29-33.

594. SAVOY-MOORE, R.T., SCHWARTZ, N.B., DUNCAN, J.A., and MAR-
      SHALL, J.C. (1981) 'Pituitatry gonadotropin-releasing
      hormone receptors on proestrus: Effect of pentobarbital
      blockade of ovulation in the rat.' Endocrinology, 109,
      1360-1364.

595. SCHRIEFERS, H., OCKENFELS, H., and PAULINI, K. (1979) 'Hydroxy-
      lation of testosterone and induction of steroid hydroxy-
      lases by pentobarbital in genetically obese mice.' [In
      German.] Arzneimittel-Forschung, 29, 292-293.

596. SHAHIDI, N.T., and BROCKS, S.M. (1972) 'Barbiturate effect in
      androgen therapy.' New England Journal of Medicine, 287,
      309.

597. SIEGEL, H.I., BAST, J.D., and GREENWALD, G.S. (1976) 'The
      effects of phenobarbital and gonadal steroids on periovula-
      tory serum levels of luteinizing hormone and follicle-
      stimulating hormone in the hamster.' Endocrinology, 98,
      48-55.

598. SILVERMAN, A.P. (1966) 'Barbiturates, lysergic acid diethylamide,
      and the social behaviour of laboratory rats.' Psychopharma-
      cologia, 10, 155-171.

599. SORRENTINO, S. (1975) 'Ovulation in PMS-treated rats with
      gonadotropin releasing hormone after pentobarbital and
      melatonin block.' Neuroendocrinology, 19, 170-176.

600. SOUTHREN, A.L., GORDON, G.G., TOCHIMOTO, S., KRIKUN, E.,
      KRIEGER, D., JACOBSON, M., and KUNTZMAN, R. (1969) 'Effect
      of n-phenylbarbital (phetharbital) on the metabolism of tes-
      tosterone and cortisol in man.' Journal of Clinical
      Endocrinology and Metabolism, 29, 251-256.

601. STETSON, M.H., and WATSON-WHITMYRE, M. (1977) 'The neural clock
      regulating estrous cyclicity in hamsters: Gonadotropin
      release following barbiturate blockade.' Biology of
      Reproduction, 16, 536-542.

602. TERASAWA, E., GOLDFOOT, D.A., and DAVIS, G.A. (1976) 'Pento-
      barbital inhibition of progesterone-induced behavioral
      estrus in ovariectomized guinea pigs.' Brain Research,
      107, 275-383.

603. TERASAWA, E., KING, M.K., WIEGAND, S.J., BRIDSON, W.E., and
      GOY, R.W. (1979) 'Barbiturate anesthesia blocks the
      positive feedback effect of progesterone, but not of
      estrogen, on luteinizing hormone release in ovariectomized
      guinea pigs.' Endocrinology, 104, 687-692.

604. TERASAWA, E., NOONAN, J., and BRIDSON, W.E. (1982) 'Anaesthesia
      with pentobarbitone blocks the progesterone-induced
      luteinizing hormone surge in the ovariectomized rhesus
      monkey.' Journal of Endocrinology, 92, 327-339.

605. TER-HAAR, M.B., and MAC KINNON, P.C. (1976) 'Effects of sodium
      pentobarbitone on serum gonadotrophin levels and on the
      incorporation of 35S from methionine into protein in the
      brain and anterior pituitary during the oestrous cycle of
      the rat.' Journal of Endocrinology, 68, 289-296.

606. TERRANOVA, P.F. (1980) 'Effects of phenobarbital-induced ovula-
      tory delay on the follicular population and serum levels of
      steroids and gonadotropins in the hamster: A model for
      atresia.' Biology of Reproduction, 23, 92-99.

607. TYLER, J.L., and GORSKI, R.A. (1980) 'Temporal limits for
      copulation-induced ovulation in the pentobarbital-blocked
      proestrous rat.' Endocrinology, 106, 1815-1819.

608. UNGERER, J.C., HARFORD, R.J., and BROWN, T.L. (1976) 'Sex
      guilt and preferences for illegal drugs among drug abusers.'
      Journal of Clinical Psychology, 32, 891-895.

609. VAN DER SCHOOT, P. (1978) 'Plasma oestradiol and delayed ovu-
      lation after administration of sodium pentobarbitone to
      prooestrous 5 day cyclic rats.' Journal of Endocrinology,
      77, 325-332.

610. VAN DER SCHOOT, P. (1980) 'Delay of ovulation in rats with
      sodium pentobarbitone: Apparent differences between rats
      with 4- or 5-day reproductive cycles.' Journal of Endo-
      crinology, 86, 451-457.

611. WHITLOCK, F.A. (1970) 'The syndrome of barbiturate dependence.'
      Medical Journal of Australia, 2, 391-396.

612. WISE, P.M., RANCE, N., SELMANOFF, M., and BARRACLOUGH, C.A.
      (1981) 'Changes in radioimmunoassayable luteinizing hormone-
      releasing hormone in discrete brain areas of the rat at
      various times on proestrus, diestrous day 1, and after
      phenobarbital administration.' Endocrinology, 108, 2179-
      2185.

613. WUTTKE, W., and MEITES, J. (1970) 'Effects of ether and pen-
      tobarbital on serum prolactin and LH levels in proestrous
      rats.' Proceedings of the Society for Experimental Biology
      and Medicine, 135, 648-652.

614. YING, S., and MEYER, R.K. (1969) 'Effect of coitus on bar-
      biturate-blocked ovulation in immature rats.' Fertility
      and Sterility, 20, 772-778.

615. YOKOYAMA, A., TOMOGANE, H., and OTA, K. (1971) 'Prolactin
      surge on the afternoon of pro-oestrus in the rat and its
      blockade by pentobarbitone.' Experientia, 27, 578-579.

616.   ZAIDI, P., WICKINGS, E.J., and NIESCHLAS, E.   (1982)   'The effects
       of ketamine HCl and barbiturate anaesthesia on the metabolic
       clearance and production rates of testosterone in the
       male rhesus monkey, Macaca mulatta.'   Journal of Steroid
       Biochemistry, 16, 463-466.

617.   ZEILMAKER, G.H., and MOLL, J.   (1967)   'Effects of progesterone
       and pentobarbitone on hypothalamic induction of ovulation
       in the 5-day cyclic rat.'   Acta Endocrinologica, 55, 378-388.

Benzodiazepines

618. ANSARI, J.M. (1976) 'Impotence: Prognosis (a controlled
      study).' British Journal of Psychiatry, 128, 194-198.

619. ARGUELLES, A.E., and ROSNER, J. (1975) 'Diazepam and plasma-
      testosterone levels.' [Letter.] Lancet, 2, 607.

620. BAILEY, H.R. (1973) 'Studies in depression. II. Treatment of
      the depressed, frigid woman.' Medical Journal of Aus-
      tralia, 1, 834-837.

621. BARTH, C. (1968) 'The treatment of psycho-autonomic syndromes
      in a gynecological outpatient department with Limbatril.'
      [In German.] Münchener Medizinische Wochenschrift, 110,
      2525-2527.

622. BERGMAN, D., FUTTERWEIT, W., SEGAL, R., and SIROTA, D. (1981)
      'Increased oestradiol in diazepam related gynaecomastia.'
      [Letter.] Lancet, 2, 1225-1226.

623. BERTONE, C., and CANNELLA, M. (1971) 'Treatment of the climac-
      teric syndrome: Clinical data on the use of the association
      of chlordiazepoxide and conjugated estrogens (Menrium).'
      [In Italian.] Minerva Ginecologia, 23, 902-906.

624. BORZECKI, Z., REJOWSKA, J., JARZEBOWSKI, E., and SWIES, Z.
      (1979) 'The influence of oxazepam and diazepam on the
      sexual behaviour and level of GABA biogenic amines in a
      male rat's brain.' Annales Universitatis Mariae Curie-
      Sklodowska, Sectio D: Medicina, 34, 371-376.

625. BROWN, R.S., MAZANSKY, H., and MAXWELL, H.M. (1968) 'Priapism.'
      South African Medical Journal, 42, 886-889.

626. CAHN, B. (1966) 'Electrolyte and hormonal balance in human
      subjects following diazepam administration.' Current
      Therapeutic Research, Clinical and Experimental, 8, 256-
      260.

627. CARTER, C.S., DAILY, R.F., and LEAF, R. (1977) 'Effects of chlordiazepoxide, oxazepam, chlorpromazine, and D-amphetamine on sexual responses in male and female hamsters.' Psychopharmacology, 55, 195-201.

628. CHETANASILPIN, P., TUCHINDA, P., and CHENPANICH, K. (1975) 'Effects of some drugs on psychosexual response in man.' Journal of the Medical Association of Thailand, 58, 509-514.

629. COBO, M.S., RAMIREZ, C.T., and BONET, H.M. (1975) 'Use of lorazepam in the menopause, sterility, frigidity, and obesity.' [In Spanish.] Ginecologia y Obstetricia de Mexico, 37, 305-310.

630. COCCHI, R., and GHIGLIONE-ROCCA, R. (1977) 'Neurotic masturbation and infantile depression: Clinico-terapeutic approach and possible peuro-psychological explanation.' [In Italian.] Acta Neurologica, 32, 229-241.

631. COOK, P.S., NOTELOVITZ, M., KALRA, P.S., and KALRA, S.P. (1979) 'Effect of diazepam on serum testosterone and the ventral prostate gland in male rats.' Archives of Andrology, 3, 31-35.

632. COPER, H. (1969) 'Sexual disorders induced by Valium.' Deutsche Medizinische Wochenschrift, 94, 1467.

633. ELSDON-DEW, R.W. (1975) 'Clinical trials of oxprenolol in anxiety.' Scottish Medical Journal, 29, 286-287.

634. ERKKOLA, R., IISALO, E., and PUNNONEN, R. (1973) 'The effect of propranolol and oxazepam on some vegetative menopausal symptoms.' Annals of Clinical Research, 5, 208-213.

635. ESSMAN, W.B. (1978) 'Benzodiazepines and aggressive behavior.' Modern Problems of Pharmacopsychiatry, 13, 13-28.

636. FIGLER, M.H., KLEIN, R.M., and THOMPSON, C.S. (1975) 'Chlordiazepoxide (Librium)-induced changes in intraspecific attack and selected non-agonistic behaviors in male Siamese fighting fish.' Psychopharmacologia, 42, 139-145.

637. FLOYD, W.S. (1971) 'Psychopharmacological estrogen activity.' Behavioral Neuropsychiatry, 3, 22-24.

638. FONTANA, A. (1970) 'Results of the action of a limbicotropic drug on 100 hyposocial subjects of developmental age: Preliminary note.' [In Italian.] Minerva Pediatrica, 22, 448-452.

639. FOX, K.A., and GUERRIERO, F.J. (1978) 'Effect of benzodiazepines on age of vaginal perforation and first estrus in mice.' Research Communications in Psychology, Psychiatry, and Behavior, 21, 181-184.

640. GAILLARD, J.M., and PHELIPPEAU, M. (1976) 'Benzodiazepine-
          induced modifications of dream content: The effect of
          flunitrazepam.' Neuropsychobiology, 2, 37-44.

641. GORDON, L.A., MOSTOFSKY, D.I., and GORDON, G.G. (1980)
          'Changes in testosterone levels in the rat following intra-
          peritoneal cocaine HCl.' International Journal of Neuro-
          science, 11, 139-141.

642. GRANDISON, L. (1982) 'Suppression of prolactin secretion by
          benzodiazepines in vivo.' Neuroendocrinology, 34, 369-373.

643. GREENBLATT, D.J., and SHADER, R.I. (1974) Benzodiazepines in
          Clinical Practice. New York: Raven Press.

644. HALBERSTADT, E., and TAUBERT, H.D. (1968) 'Management of
          climacteric disorders using a new combination drug Menrium.'
          [In German.] Medizinische Klinik, 63, 1229-1231.

645. HEINEN, G. (1968) 'Influencing the endometrium and vaginal
          epithelium through the administration of conjugated estro-
          genic substances in combination with a psychopharmacologic
          agent.' [In German.] Medizinische Welt, 27, 1585-1588.

646. HORSKY, J. (1979) 'Effect of natural estrogens and diazepam
          alone and in combination on the climacteric syndrome.'
          Münchener Medizinische Wochenschrift, 121, 765-766.

647. HUGHES, J.M. (1964) 'Failure to ejaculate with chlordiazepox-
          ide.' American Journal of Psychiatry, 121, 610-611.

648. JOEL, C.A. (1972) 'Pathogenesis, diagnosis, and treatment of
          impotentia coeundi with special reference to hyperzoospermia
          and therapy with diazepine-derivative.' Andrologie, 4,
          7-14.

649. KHAN, A.A. (1980) 'Preliminary in vitro study of diazepam and
          droperidol on oestrus rat uterus.' British Journal of
          Anaesthesia, 52, 349-354.

650. KURLAND, A.A., BETHON, G.D., MICHAUX, M.H., and AGALLIANOS, D.D.
          (1966) 'Chlorpromazine-chlordiazepoxide and chlorproamize-
          imipramine treatment: Side effects and clinical laboratory
          findings.' Journal of New Drugs, 6, 80-95.

651. LEAVITT, F. (1969) 'Drug-induced modifications in sexual behav-
          ior and open field locomotion of male rats.' Physiology and
          Behavior, 4, 677-683.

652. MAISS, H.J. (1968) 'Therapy of psycho-autonomic and dysphoric
          syndromes in the general practice.' [In German.] Med-
          izinische Klinik, 63, 727-730.

653. MANEKSHA, S., and HARRY, T.V. (1975) 'Lorazepam in sexual
          disorders.' British Journal of Clinical Practice, 29,
          175-176.

654. MC CLAIN, R.M., and HOAR, R.M. (1980) 'The effect of flunitra-
      zepam on reproduction in the rat: The use of cross-foster-
      ing in the evaluation of postnatal parameters in rat repro-
      duction studies.' Toxicology and Applied Pharmacology, 53,
      92-100.

655. MILLS, L.C. (1975) 'Drug-induced impotence.' American Family
      Physician, 12, 104-106.

656. SCHWARTZ, E.D., and SMITH, J.J. (1963) 'The effect of chlor-
      diazepoxide on the female reproductive cycle as tested in
      infertility patients.' Western Journal of Surgery in
      Obstetrics and Gynecology, 71, 74-76.

657. SIERRA, G., ACUNA, C., OTERO, J., and COCAMPO, G. (1969) 'Ex-
      perimental study of a new psychosedative drug: HS-2314.'
      International Journal of Neuropharmacology, 8, 153-160.

658. SIMIONESCU, S., BORDEIANU, A., STANCU, C., DANIEL, B., PINTILES-
      CU, V., MATEESCU-CANTUNIARI, A., and MATEESCUAACANTUNIARI, A.
      (1974) 'The nonspecific pharmacodynamic action of certain
      psychotropic drugs of different structure and classification
      on the equilibrium of sexual function.' Revue Roumaine de
      Physiologie, 11, 253-263.

659. USDIN, G.L. (1960) 'Preliminary report on librium, a new
      psychopharmacologic agent.' Journal of the Louisiana State
      Medical Society, 112, 142-147.

660. VERRELLI, D., MANSANI, F.E., and CAVATORIA, E. (1974) 'Combin-
      ation of natural estrogens and anxiolytic drugs in meno-
      pausal disturbances.' Minerva Ginecologica, 26, 351-357.

661. WHITELAW, M.J. (1961) 'Menstrual irregularities associated with
      use of methaminodiazepoxide.' Journal of the American
      Medical Association, 175, 400-401.

662. WILKINSON, M., MOGER, W.H., and GROVESTINE, D. (1980) 'Chronic
      treatment with Valium (diazepam) fails to affect the
      reproductive system of the male rat.' Life Sciences, 27,
      2285-2291.

663. WILLIAMSON, R.A., and STENCHEVER, M.A. (1981) 'The effect of
      diazepam on rates of fertilization in the CF-1 mouse.'
      American Journal of Obstetrics and Gynecology, 139, 178-
      181.

664. ZIEMANN, H., and LUDWIG, H. (1969) 'The effect of Menrium on
      the vaginal cell picture in female castrates and the in-
      fluencing of so-called climacteric disorders.' [In German.]
      Medizinische Welt, 28, 1571-1574.

Caffeine

665. BUNGE, R. G. (1973) 'Caffeine-stimulation of ejaculated human
      spermatozoa.' Urology, 1, 371-375.

666. BARKAY, J., ZUCKERMAN, H., SKLAN, D., and GORDON, S. (1977)
      'Effect of caffeine on increasing the motility of
      frozen human sperm.' Fertility and Sterility, 28,
      175-179.

667. GARBERS, D. L., FIRST, N. L., SULLIVAN, J. J., and LARDY, H. A.
      (1971) 'Stimulation and maintenace of ejaculated bovine
      spermatozoan respiration and motility by caffeine.'
      Biology of Reproduction, 5, 336-341.

667a GARBERS, D. L., LUST, W. D., FIRST, N. L., and LARDY, H. A.
      (1971) 'Effects of phosphodiesterase inhibitors and
      cyclic nucleotides on sperm respiration and motility.'
      Biochemistry, 10, 1825-1830.

667b HARRISON, R. F. (1978) 'Insemination of husband's semen with
      and without the addition of caffeine.' Fertility
      and Sterility, 29, 532-536.

667c HAESUNGCHARRERN, A., and CHULAVATNATAL, M. (1973) 'Stimulation
      of human spermatozoal motility by caffeine.'
      Fertility and Sterility, 24, 662-666.

667d SCHOENFELD, C., AMELAR, R. D., and DUBIN, L. (1975)
      'Stimulation of ejaculated human spermatozoa by caffeine.'
      Fertility and Sterility, 26, 158-165.

667e ZIMBARDO, P., and BARRY, H. (1958) 'Effects of caffeine
      and chlorpromazine in the sexual behavior of male rats.'
      Science, 127, 84-85.

Cocaine

668. ANONYMOUS. (1925) 'Cocainism and homosexuality.' Journal of the American Medical Association, 85, 1936.

669. ASHLEY, R. (1975) 'Cocaine: Its history, uses, and effects.' New York: St. Martin's Press.

670. BEJARANO, J. (1952) 'Further considerations on the coca habit in Colombia.' Bulletin on Narcotics, 4, 3-19.

671. BELL, D.S. (1971) 'The precipitants of amphetamine addiction.' British Journal of Psychiatry, 119, 171-179.

672. BYCK, R., and VAN DYKE, C. (1977) 'What are the effects of cocaine in man?' In: P.C. Peterson and R.C. Stillman, eds. Cocaine: 1977. Rockville, maryland: NIDA Research Monograph, pp. 97-112.

673. CARROLL, E. (1977) 'Coca: The plant and its use.' In: P.C. Peterson and R.C. Stillman, eds. Cocaine: 1977. Rockville, Maryland: NIDA Research Monograph.

674. CHOPRA, R., and CHOPRA, G. (1930/31) 'Cocaine habit in India.' Indian Journal of Medical Research, 18, 1013-1046.

675. CHOPRA, R., and CHOPRA, I. (1957) 'Treatment of drug addiction: Experience in India.' Bulletin on Narcotics, 9, 21-33.

676. COHEN, S. (1975) 'Cocaine.' Journal of the American Medical Association, 231, 74-75.

677. CROWLEY, A. (1922) Diary of a Drug Fiend. London: William Collins Sons.

678. DANIEL, E.E., and WOLOWYK, M. (1966) 'The contractile response of the uterus to cocaine.' Canadian Journal of Physiology and Pharmacology, 44, 721-730.

679. DU PONT, R.L.   (1982)   'Problems of using cocaine as an aphro-
      disiac.'   Medical Aspects of Human Sexuality, 6, 14.

680. EBERLE, E.G., and GORDON, F.T.   (1903)   'Report of the committee
      on the acquirement of drug habits.'   American Journal of
      Pharmacy, 75, 474-485.

681. FAVILLI, M.   (1951)   'Stato psichico nill'ebbrezza der cocaina.'
      ['The psychic state in cocaine inebriety.']   Rasse di Studi
      Psichiatrici, 40, 740-747.

682. FREUD, S.   (1974)   Cocaine Papers.   Stonehill, New York.

683. GAY, G.R.   (1981)   'You've come a long way, baby!   Coke time
      for the new American lady of the lights.'   Journal of
      Psychoactive Drugs, 13, 297-318.

684. GAY, G.R., NEWMEYER, J.A., ELION, R.A., and WIEDER, S.   (1975)
      'Drug-sex practice in the Haight-Ashbury or "the sensuous
      hippie."'   In: M. Sandler and G.L. Gessa, eds.   Sexual
      Behavior: Pharmacology and Biochemistry.   New York:
      Raven Press, pp. 63-79.

685. GAY, G.R., NEWMEYER, J.A., PERRY, M., JOHNSON, G., and KURLAND,
      M.   (1982)   'Love and Haight: The sensuous hippie revis-
      ited.'   Drug/sex practices in San Francisco 1980-1981.'
      Journal of Psychoactive Drugs, 14, 111-123.

686. GAY, G.R., SHEPPARD, C.W., INABA, D.S., and NEWMEYER, J.A.
      (1973)   'An old girl--Flyin' low, dyin' slow: Cocaine in
      perspective.'   International Journal of the Addictions,
      8, 1027-1042.

687. GAY, G.R., and SMITH, D.E.   (1973)   'A free clinic approach to
      to drug abuse.'   Preventive Medicine, 2, 543-553.

688. GRINSPOON, L., and BAKALAR, J.B.   (1976)   Cocaine: A Drug and
      Its Social Evolution.   New York: Basic Books.

689. GUTIERREZ-NORIEGA, C.   (1944)   'Accion de la coca sobre la
      actividad mental de sujetos habituados.'   ['Action of
      cocaine on mental activity of habitual subjects.']   Revista
      de Medicina Experimental, 3, 1-18.

690. GUTTIERREZ-NORIEGA, C.   (1947)   'Alteraciones mentales pro-
      oudecas por la coca.'   ['Mental alterations proceeding from
      coca.']   Revista de Neuro-Psiquiatria, 10, 145-176.

691. HARTMANN, H.   (1928)   'Kokainismus und Homosexualität.'   ['Co-
      cainism and homosexuality.']   Deutsche Medizinische Wochen-
      schrift, 54, 268-270.

692. JAEL, E., and FRANKEL, F.   (1924)   Der Cocainismus: Ein Bei-
      trag zur Geschichte und Psychopathologie der Rauschgifte.
      [Cocainism: A Contribution to the History and Psycho-
      pathology of Drugs.]   Berlin: Springer Verlag.

693. JERI, F.R., SANCHEZ, C., DEL POZO, T., and FERNANDEZ, M. (1978)
     'The syndrome of coca paste.' Journal of Psychedelic
     Drugs, 10, 361-370.

694. KOLB, R. (1962) Drug Addiction: A Medical Problem. Spring-
     field, Illinois: Charles C. Thomas.

695. MAIER, H.W. (1926) Der Kokainismus. [Cocainism.] Leipzig:
     Geng Thieme.

696. MAYER-GROSS, W., SLATER, E., and ROTH, M. (1960) Clinical
     Psychiatry. Baltimore, Maryland: Williams and Williams.

697. MIRIN, S.M. (1982) 'Adverse sexual effects of cocaine.'
     Medical Aspects of Human Sexuality, 16, 13-14.

698. NAIL, R.L., GUNDERSON, E., and KOLB, D. (1974) 'Motives for
     drug use among light and heavy users.' Journal of Nervous
     and Mental Disease, 149, 131-136.

699. NEWMEYER, J.A. (1975) 'Gay-straight differences in regard to
     drugs and sexuality.' Drug Forum, 5.

700. NEWMEYER, J.A. (1978) 'The current status of cocaine use in
     San Francisco Bay area.' In: A. Schechter, ed. Drug
     Abuse, Modern Trends, Issues, and Perspectives. New York:
     Marcel Dekker.

701. OLDEN, M. (1973) Cocaine. New York: Lancer Books.

702. SANTAGELO, G. (1930) 'Le alterazioni del carattere nel
     cocainismo cronica.' ['Character alterations in chronic
     cocainism.'] Archivio Generale de Neurologia e Psichiatria,
     11, 296-306.

703. SIEGEL, R.K. (1977) 'Cocaine: Recreational use and intox-
     ication.' In: P.C. Peterson and R.C. Stillman, eds.
     Cocaine: 1977. Rockville, Maryland: NIDA Research
     Monograph Series, Volume 13, pp. 119-136.

704. SIEGEL, R.K. (1982) 'Cocaine and sexual dysfunction: The
     curse of mama coca.' Journal of Psychedelic Drugs, 14,
     71-74.

705. SPOTTS, J.V., and SHORTZ, F.C. (1980) Cocaine Users: A Repre-
     sentative Case Approach. New York: Free Press.

706. UNGERER, J., HARFORD, R., BROWN, F., and KLEBER, H. (1976)
     'Sex guilt and preferences for illegal drugs among drug
     abusers.' Journal of Clinical Psychology, 32, 891-895.

707. VERVAECK, L. (1923) 'Quelques aspects médicaux et psycho-
     logiques de la cocainomanie.' ['Several medical and psycho-
     logical aspects of cocaine mania.'] Le Scapel, 76, 744.

708. VON SCHEIDT, J. (1973) 'Sigmund Freud und das Kokain.'
      ['Sigmund Freud and cocaine.'] Psyche, 27, 385-430.

709. WALDORF, D., MURPHY, S., REINERMAN, C., and BRIDGET, J. (1977)
      'Doing coke: An ethnography of cocaine users and sellers.'
      Washington, D.C.: Drug Abuse Council, pp. 16-68.

710. WESSON, D.R. (1982) 'Use of cocaine by masseuses.' Journal
      of Psychoactive Drugs, 14, 75-76.

711. WESSON, D.R., and SMITH, D.E. (1977) 'Cocaine: Its use for
      central nervous system stimulation including recreational
      and medical uses.' In: P.C. Peterson and R.C. Stillman,
      eds. Cocaine: 1977. Washington, D.C.: U.S. Government
      Printing Office, NIDA Research Monograph No. 13, pp. 137-
      152.

712. WINICK, C., and KINSIE, P. (1971) The Lively Commerce: Pros-
      titution in the United States. Chicago, Illinois: Quad-
      rangle Books.

713. WOLFF, P. (1932) 'Drug addiction--a worldwide problem.'
      Journal of the American Medical Association, 98, 175-184.

714. ALEXANDER, M. (1967) The Sexual Paradise of LSD. North
          Hollywood: Brandon House.

715. ALPERT, R. (1969) 'Drugs and sexual behavior.' Journal
          of Sex Research, 5, 50-56.

716. ALPERT, R. (1969) 'LSD and sexuality.' Psychedelic Review,
          10, 21-24.

717. ARONSON, B., and OSMOND, H. (1970) Psychedelics. Garden
          City, New York: Doubleday Co.

718. BALL, J.R., and ARMSTRONG, J.J. (1961) 'The use of LSD in
          the treatment of sexual perversions.' Canadian Psychiatric
          Association Journal, 6, 231.

719. BIGNAMI, G. (1966) 'Pharmacological influences on mating
          behavior in the male rat.' Psychopharmacology, 10,
          44-58.

720. COHEN, S. (1960) 'Lysergic acid diethylamide: Side effects
          and complications.' Journal of Nervous and Mental
          Disease, 130, 30.

721. DAHLBERG, C.C. (1971) 'Sexual behavior in the drug culture.'
          Medical Aspects of Human Sexuality, 5, 64-71.

722. FREEDMAN, A.M. (1967) 'Drugs and sexual behavior.' Medical
          Aspects of Human Sexuality, 1, 25-31.

723. GELLER, A., and BOAS, M. (1969) The Drug Beat. New York:
          Cowles Book Co.

724. GILLETT, E. (1960) 'Effects of chlorpromazine and D-lysergic
          acid diethylamide on sex behavior of male rats.'
          Proceedings of the Society of Experimental Biology and
          Medicine, 103, 392-394.

725. GIOSCIA, V. (1969) 'LSD subcultures: Acidoxy verses
          orthodoxy.' American Journal of Orthopsychiatry,
          39, 428-429.

726. GROF, S. (1975) Realms of the Human Unconscious: Obser-
          vations From LSD Research. New York: Viking Press.

727. HENSALA, J., EPSTEIN, L., and BLACKEN, K. (1967) 'LSD and
          psychiatric inpatients.' Archives of General Psychiatry,
          16, 554-559.

728. LEARY, T. (1970) The Politics of Ecstasy. New York:
          G. Putnam's Sons.

729. SOULAIRAC, M. (1963) 'Etude experimentale des regulations
          hormononerveuses du compartment sexual du rat male.'
          Annales D'Endocrinologie, 24, 1-98.

730. SOULAIRAC, M.L., and SOULAIRAC, A. (1975) 'Monoaminergic
          and cholingeric control of sexual behavior in the male
          rat.' In: M. Sandler and G.L. Gessa, eds. Sexual
          Behavior: Pharmacology and Biochemistry. New York:
          Raven Press, pp. 99-116.

731. STAFFORD, P., and GOLIGHTLY, B. (1967) LSD: The Problem-
          Solving Psychedelic. New York: Award Books.

732. THORNE, M.G.,JR., and SALES, B. (1967) 'Marital and LSD
          therapy with a transvestite and his wife.' Journal of
          Sex Research, 3, 169-177.

733. WAKEFIELD, D. (1964) 'A reporter's objective view.' In:
          D. Solomon, ed. LSD: The Consciousness-Expanding Drug.
          New York: G. P. Putnam's Sons.

734. ZENTNER, J.L. (1976) 'The recreational use of LSD-25 and
          drug prohibition.' Journal of Psychedelic Drugs, 8,
          299-303.

735. ABEL, E.L. (1976) The Scientific Study of Marihuana.
      Chicago: Nelson-Hall.

736. ABEL, E.L. (1980) Marihuana: The First Twelve Thousand Years.
      New York: Plenum Press.

737. ABEL, E.L. (1981) 'Marihuana and sex: A critical survey.'
      Drug and Alcohol Dependence, 8, 1-22.

738. ALDRICH, M.R. (1977) 'Tantric cannabis use in India.' Journal
      of Psychedelic Drugs, 9, 227-233.

739. AMENDT, G. (1974) 'Haschisch und Sexualität--eine empirische
      Untersuchung über die Sexualität jugendlicher in der
      Drogensubkultur.' Beiträge zur Sexualforschung, 53, 1-124.

740. ANONYMOUS. (1975) 'Marihuana and testosterones: A discussion.'
      In: J.R. Tinklenberg, ed. Marihuana and Health Hazards:
      Methodological Issues in Current Research. New York:
      Academic Press, pp. 95-101.

741. ARAFAT, I., and YORBURG, B. (1972) 'Drug use and the sexual
      behaviour of college women.' Journal of Sex Research, 9,
      21-29.

742. ASCH, R.H., FERNANDEZ, E.O., SMITH, C.G., and PAUERSTEIN, C.J.
      (1979) 'Precoital single doses of delta-9-tetrahydro-
      cannabinol block ovulation in the rabbit.' Fertility and
      Sterility, 31, 331-   .

743. AYALON, D., NIR, I., CORDOVA, T., BAUMINGER, S., PUDER, M.,
      NAOR, Z., KASHI, R., ZOR, U., HARELL, A., and LINDNER, H.R.
      (1977) 'Acute effect of delta-1-tetrahydrocannabinol on
      the hypothalamo-pituitary-ovarian axis in the rat.'
      Neuroendocrinology, 23, 31-43.

744. BESCH, N.F., SMITH, C.G., BESCH, P.K., and KAUFMAN, R.H. (1977) 'The effect of marihuana (delta-9-tetrahydrocannabinol) on the secretion of luteinizing hormone in the ovariectomized rhesus monkey.' American Journal of Obstetrics and Gynecology, 128, 635- .

745. BLOCH, E., THYSEN, B., MORRILL, G.A., GARDNER, E., and FUJIMOTO, G. (1978) 'Effects of cannabinoids on reproduction and development.' Vitamins and Hormones, 36, 203-258.

746. BLOOMQUIST, E.R. (1968) Marijuana. Beverly Hills, California: Gencoe Press.

747. BORGEN, L.A., LOTT, G.C., and DAVIS, M. (1973) 'Cannabis-induced hypothermia: A dose-effect comparison of crude marihuana extract and synthetic delta-9-tetrahydrocannbinol in male and female rats.' Research Communications in Chemical Pathology and Pharmacology, 5, 621-626.

748. BOUQUET, J. (1951) 'Cannabis. III. Cannabis intoxication.' Bulletin on Narcotics, 3, 22.

749. BROMLEY, B.L., RABII, J., GORDON, J.H., and ZIMMERMAN, E. (1978) 'Delta-9-tetrahydrocannabinol inhibition of suckling-induced prolactin release in the lactating rat.' Endocrine Research Communications, 5, 271-278.

750. BURDSAL, C., GREENBERG, G., BELL, M., and REYNOLDS, S. (1975) 'A factor-analytic examination of sexual behaviors and attitudes and marihuana usage.' Journal of Clinical Psychology, 31, 568-572.

751. BURSTEIN, S., HUNTER, S.A., and SHOUPE, T.S. (1979) 'Cannabinoid inhibition of rat luteal cell progesterone synthesis.' Research Communications in Chemical Pathology and Pharmacology, 24, 413-416.

752. BURSTEIN, S., HUNTER, S.A., and SHOUPE, T.S. (1979) 'Site of inhibition of Leydig cell testosterone synthesis by delta-1-tetrahydrocannabinol.' Molecular Pharmacology, 15, 633-640.

753. BURSTEIN, S., HUNTER, S.A., SHOUPE, T.S., TAYLOR, P., BARTKE, A., and DALTERIO, S. (1978) 'Cannabinoid inhibition of testosterone synthesis by mouse Leydig cells.' Research Communications in Chemical Pathology and Pharmacology, 19, 557-560.

754. BURSTEIN, S., LEVIN, E., and VARANELLI, C. (1973) 'Prostaglandins and cannabis. II. Inhibition of biosynthesis by the naturally occurring cannabinoids.' Biochemical Pharmacology, 22, 2905-2910.

755. BURSTEIN, S., and RAZ, A. (1972) 'Inhibition of prostaglandin E$_2$ biosynthesis by delta-1-tetrahydrocannabinol.' Prostaglandins, 2, 369-374.

756. BUYS, D. (1979) 'Pot smoking by pregnant women may be hazardous.' U.S. Journal, July, 8.

757. CATES, W., JR., and POPE, J.N. (1977) 'Gynecomastia and cannabis smoking.' American Journal of Surgery, 134, 613-615.

758. CHAKRAVARTY, I., and GHOSH, J.J. (1981) 'Influence of cannabis and delta-9-tetrahydrocannabinol on the biochemistry of the male reproductive organs.' Biochemical Pharmacology, 30, 273-276.

759. CHAKRAVARTY, I., SENGUPTA, D., BHATTACHARYYA, P., and GHOSH, J.J. (1975) 'Effect of treatment with cannabis extract on the water and glycogen contents of the uterus in normal and estradiol-treated prepubertal rats.' Toxicology and Applied Pharmacology, 34, 513-516.

760. CHAKRAVARTY, I., SHAH, P.G., SHETH, A.R., and GHOSH, J.J. (1979) 'Mode of action of delta-9-tetrahydrocannabinol on hypothalamo-pituitary function in adult female rats.' Journal of Reproduction and Fertility, 57, 113-117.

761. CHAKRAVARTY, I., SHETH, A.R., and GHOSH, J.J. (1975) 'Effect of acute delta-9-tetrahydrocannabinol treatment on serum luteinizing hormone and prolactin levels in adult female rats.' Fertility and Sterility, 26, 947-948.

762. CHAKRAVARTY, I., SHETH, P.R., SHETH, A.R., and GHOSH, J.J. (1982) 'Delta-9-tetrahydrocannabinol: Its effect on hypotalamo-pituitary system in male rats.' Archives of Andrology, 8, 25-27.

763. CHAN, M.Y., and TSE, A. (1978) 'The effect of cannabinoids (delta-9-THC and delta-8-THC) on hepatic microsomal metabolism of testosterone in vitro.' Biochemical Pharmacology, 27, 1725-1728.

764. CHAUSOW, A.M., and SAPER, C.B. (1974) 'Marihuana and sex.' New England Journal of Medicine, 291, 308.

765. CHOPRA, G. (1969) 'Man and marijuana.' International Journal of the Addictions, 4, 215-247.

766. COHEN, M., and KLEIN, D. (1970) 'Drug abuse in a young psychiatric population.' American Journal of Orthopsychiatry, 40, 448-455.

767. COHEN, S. (1975) 'The sex-pot controversy.' Drug Abuse and Alcoholism Newsletter, 4, 1-4.

768. COHEN, S. (1982) 'Cannabis and sex: Multifaceted paradoxes.'
      Journal of Psychoactive Drugs, 14, 55-58.

769. COHEN, S. (1982) 'Patterns of lethal drug abuse and sexuality.'
      Medical Aspects of Human Sexuality, 16, 132-137.

770. COHEN, R.A., BARRATT, E.S., and PIRCH, J.H. (1974) 'Marijuana
      responses in rats: Influence of castration or testosterone
      (38053).' Proceedings of the Society for Experimental
      Biology and Medicine, 146, 109-113.

771. COLLU, R. (1976) 'Endocrine effects of chronic intraventricular
      administration of delta-9-tetrahydrocannabinol to prepuber-
      al and adult male rats.' Life Sciences, 18, 223-230.

772. COLLU, R., LETARTE, J., LEBOEUF, G., and DUCHARME, J.R. (1975)
      'Endocrine effects of chronic administration of psychoactive
      drugs to prepuberal male rats.' Life Sciences, 16, 533-542.

773. COOPER, C.R. (1937) Here's to Crime. Boston, Massachusetts:
      Little, Brown, and Co.

774. COPELAND, K.C., UNDERWOOD, L.E., and VAN WYK, J.J. (1980)
      'Marihuana smoking and puberal arrest.' Journal of Ped-
      iatrics, 96, 1079-1080.

775. CORCORAN, M.E., AMIT, Z., MALSBURY, C.W., and DAYKIN, S. (1974)
      'Reduction in copulatory behavior of male rats following
      hashish injections.' Research Communications in Chemical
      Pathology and Pharmacology, 7, 779-782.

776. CUSHMAN, P., JR. (1975) 'Plasma testosterone levels in
      healthy male marijuana smokers. American Journal of Drug
      and Alcohol Abuse, 2, 269-275.

777. CUTLER, M.G., MACKINTOSH, J.H., and CHANCE, M.R. (1975)
      'Cannabis resin and sexual behaviour in the laboratory
      mouse.' Psychopharmacologia, 45, 129-131.

778. DALEY, J.D., BRANDA, L.A., ROSENFELD, J., and YOUNGLAI, E.V.
      (1974) 'Increase of serum prolactin in male rats by
      (-)-trans-delta-9-tetrahydrocannabinol.' Journal of
      Endocrinology, 63, 415-416.

779. DALTERIO, S. (1980) 'Perinatal or adult exposure to cannabin-
      oids alters male reproductive functions in mice.' Pharm-
      acology, Biochemistry, and Behavior, 12, 143-153.

780. DALTERIO, S., and BARTKE, A. (1979) 'Perinatal exposure to
      cannabinoids alters male reproductive function in mice.'
      Science, 205, 1420-1422.

781. DALTERIO, S., BARTKE, A., and BURSTEIN, S. (1977) 'Cannabin-
      oids inhibit testosterone secretion by mouse testes in
      vitro.' Science, 196, 1472-1473.

782.   DALTERIO, S., BARTKE, A., HARPER, M.J.K., HUFFMAN, R., and
        SWEENEY, C. (1981) 'Effects of cannabinoids and female
        exposure on the pituitary-testicular axis in mice:
        Possible involvement of prostaglandins.' Biology of
        Reproduction, 24, 315-322.

783.   DALTERIO, S., BARTKE, A., and MAYFIELD, D. (1981) 'A novel
        female influences delta-9-THC effects on plasma hormone
        levels in male mice.' Pharmacology, Biochemistry, and
        Behavior, 15, 281-284.

784.   DALTERIO, S., BARTKE, A., ROBERSON, C., WATSON, D., and BURSTEIN,
        S. (1978) 'Direct and pituitary-mediated effects of
        delta-9-THC and cannabinol on the testis.' Pharmacology,
        Biochemistry, and Behavior, 8, 673-678.

785.   DALTERIO, S., BARTKE, A., and SWEENEY, C. (1981) 'Inter-
        active effects of ethanol and delta-9-tetrahydrocannabinol
        on endocrine functions in male mice.' Journal of Andrology,
        2, 87-93.

786.   DALTERIO, S., BLUM, K., DELALLO, L., SWEENEY, C., BRIGGS, A.,
        and BARTKE, A. (1980) 'Perinatal exposure to delta-9-THC
        in mice: Altered enkephalin and norepinephrine sensi-
        tivity in vas deferens.' Substance and Alcohol Actions/Mis-
        use, 1, 467-478.

787.   DALTERIO, S., MICHAEL, S.D., MACMILLAN, B.T., and BARTKE, A.
        (1981) 'Differential effects of cannabinoid exposure and
        stress on plasma prolactin, growth hormone, and cortico-
        sterone levels in male mice.' Life Sciences, 28, 761-766.

788.   DE FARIAS, R.C. (1955) 'Use of maconha (Cannabis sativa L)
        in Brazil.' Bulletin on Narcotics, 1, 5-19.

789.   DIXIT, V.P., ARYA, M., and LOHIYA, N.K. (1975) 'The effect of
        chronically administered cannabis extract on the female
        genital tract of mice and rats.' Endokrinologie, 66,
        365-   .

790.   DIXIT, V.P., GUPTA, C.L., and AGRAWAL, M. (1977) 'Testicular
        degeneration and necrosis induced by chronic administration
        of cannabis extract in dogs.' Endokrinologie, 69, 299-305.

791.   DIXIT, V.P., and LOHIYA, N.K. (1975) 'Effects of cannabis
        extract on the response of accessory sex organs of adult
        male mice to testosterone.' Indian Journal of Physiol-
        ogy and Pharmacology, 19, 98-100.

792.   DIXIT, V.P., SHARMA, V.N., and LOHIYA, N.K. (1974) 'The effect
        of chronically administered cannabis extract on the tes-
        ticular function of mice.' European Journal of Pharmacol-
        ogy, 26, 111-116.

793.   DU PONT, R.L.   (1982)   'Adverse reactions to marihuana.'
       Medical Aspects of Human Sexuality, 16, 21.

794.   EGAN, S.M., GRAHAM, J.D.P., and LEWIS, M.J.   (1976)   'The
       uptake of tritiated delta-1-tetrahydrocannabinol by the
       isolated vas deferens of the rat.'   British Journal of
       Pharmacology, 56, 413-416.

795.   EICHEL, G.R., and TROIDEN, R.R.   (1978)   'The domestication of
       drug effects: The case of marijuana.'   Journal of Psyche-
       delic Drugs, 10, 133-136.

796.   EWING, J.A.   (1972)   'Students, sex, and marijuana.'   Medical
       Aspects of Human Sexuality, 6, 101-117.

797.   FISHER, G., and STECKLER, A.   (1974)   'Psychological effects,
       personality and behavioral changes attributed to marihuana
       use.'   International Journal of the Addictions, 9, 101.

798.   FREUDENTHAL, R.I., MARTIN, J., and WALL, M.E.   (1972)   'Distri-
       bution of delta-9-tetrahydrocannabinol in the mouse.'
       British Journal of Pharmacology, 44, 244-250.

799.   FRIEDMAN, I., and PEER, I.   (1970)   'Drug addiction among pimps
       and prostitutes in Israel.'   In: S. Shoham, ed.   Israel
       Studies in Criminology, I.   Tel Aviv: Goneh Press, pp. 141-
       175.

800.   FRIEDMAN, J.G.   (1975)   'Marihuana and testosterone levels.'
       New England Journal of Medicine, February 27, 484.

801.   FUJIMOTO, G.I., KOSTELLOW, A.B., ROSENBAUM, R., MORRILL, G.A.,
       and BLOCH, E.   (1979)   'Effects of cannabinoids on repro-
       ductive organs in the female Fischer rat.'   In: G.G. Nahas
       and W.D.M. Paton, eds.   Marihuana: Biological Effects.
       New York: Pergamon Press, p. 441-449.

802.   GAWIN, F.H.   (1978)   'Drugs and eros: Reflections on aphro-
       disiacs.'   Journal of Psychedelic Drugs, 10, 227-236.

803.   GAY, G.R., NEWMEYER, J.A., PERRY, M., JOHNSON, G., and KUR-
       LAND, M.   (1982)   'Love and Haight: The sensuous hippie
       revisited. Drug/sex practices in San Francisco, 1980-81.'
       Journal of Psychoactive Drugs, 14, 111-123.

804.   GOLDSTEIN, H., HARCLERODE, J., and NYQUIST, S.E.   (1977)   'Ef-
       fects of chronic administration of delta-9-tetrahydro-
       cannibinol and cannabidiol on rat testicular esterase iso-
       zymes.'   Life Sciences, 20, 951-954.

805.   GOODE, E.   (1972)   'Drug use and sexual activity on a college
       campus.'   American Journal of Psychiatry, 128, 1272-1276.

806.   GOODE, E.   (1972)   'Sex and marijuana.'   Sexual Behavior, 2,
       45-51.

807. GORDON, J.H., BROMLEY, B.L., GORSKI, R.A., and ZIMMERMAN, E.
      (1978) 'Delta-9-tetrahydrocannabinol enhancement of
      lordosis behavior in estrogen-treated female rats.'
      Pharmacology, Biochemistry, and Behavior, 8, 603-609.

808. HALIKAS, J., WELLER, R., and MORSE, C. (1982) 'Effects of
      regular marijuana use on sexual performance.' Journal of
      Psychoactive Drugs, 14, 59-70.

809. HARCLERODE, J. (1980) 'The effect of marijuana on reproduction
      and development.' National Institute on Drug Abuse Research
      Monograph Series, 31, 137-166.

810. HARCLERODE, J., NYQUIST, S.E., NAZAR, B., and LOWE, D. (1979)
      'Effects of cannabis on sex hormones and testicular enzymes
      of the rodent.' In: G.G. Nahas and W.D.M. Paton, eds.
      Marihuana: Biological Effects. Oxford: Pergamon Press,
      pp. 395-405.

811. HARCLERODE, J.E., SMITH, R.S., and BERGER, V.E. (1982) 'Mari-
      juana and phencyclidine and their effect through the CNS
      on the reproductive system.' Archives of Andrology, 9,
      17.

812. HARMON, J., and LIAPOULIOS, M.A. (1972) 'Gynecomastia in mari-
      huana users.' New England Journal of Medicine, 287,
      936-937.

813. HARMON, J.W., LOCKE, D., ALIAPOULIOS, M.A., and MAC INDOE, J.H.
      (1976) 'Interference with testicular development by delta-
      9-tetrahydrocannabinol.' Surgical Forum, 26, 350-352.

814. HEMBREE, W.C., NAHAS, G.G., ZEIDENBERG, P., and HUANG, H.F.S.
      (1980) 'Changes in human spermatozoa associated with high
      dose marihuana smoking.' In: G.G. Nahas and W.D.M. Paton,
      eds. Marihuana: Biological Effects. Oxford: Pergamon
      Press, pp. 429-439.

815. HEMBREE, W.C., ZEIDENBERG, P., and NAHAS, G.G. (1976) 'Mari-
      huana's effects on human gonadal function. In: G.G. Nahas,
      ed. Marihuana: Chemistry, Biochemistry, and Cellular
      Effects. New York: Springer-Verlag, pp. 521-532.

816. HERZ, S. (1970) 'Behavioral patterns in sex and drug use on
      the college campus.' Journal of the Medical Society of
      New Jersey, 67, 3-6.

817. HIGH TIMES ENCYCLOPEDIA OF RECREATIONAL DRUGS. (1978)
      High Times, New York: Stonehill Publication Co.

818. HOCHMAN, J.S., and BRILL, N.Q. (1973) 'Chronic marihuana use
      and psychosocial adaptation.' American Journal of Psy-
      chiatry, 130, 132-1 .

819. HOLDEN, C. (1976) 'House chops sex-pot probe.' Science, 192,
      450.

820. HOWES, J.F., and OSGOOD, P.F. (1976) 'Cannabinoids and the
       inhibition of prostaglandin synthesis.' In: G.G. Nahas,
       ed. Marihuana: Chemistry, Biochemistry, and Cellular
       Effects. New York: Springer-Verlag, pp. 415-424.

821. HUANG, H.F.S., NAHAS, G.G., and HEMBREE, W.C. (1980) 'Effects
       of marihuana inhalation on spermatogenesis of the rat.'
       In: G.G. Nahas and W.D.M. Paton, eds. Marihuana: Bio-
       logical Effects. Oxford: Pergamon Press, pp. 419-427.

822. HUSAIN, S., LAME, M., and DE BOER, B. (1979) 'Rat testicular
       tissue glucose metabolism in the presence of delta-9-
       cannabinol.' Proceedings of the Western Pharmacology
       Society, 22, 355-358.

823. INDIAN HEMP DRUGS COMMISSION REPORT. (1893-1894) London:
       Government Printing Office.

824. ISSIDORIDES, M.R. (1980) 'Observations in chronic hashish
       users: Nuclear aberrations in blod and sperm and abnormal
       acrosomes in spermatozoa.' In G.G. Nahas and W.D.M. Paton,
       eds. Marihuana: Biological Effects. Oxford: Pergamon
       Press, pp. 377-388.

825. JAKUBOVIC, A., and MC GEER, P.L. (1976) 'In vitro inhibition
       of protein and nucleic acid synthesis in rat testicular
       tissue by cannabinoids.' In: G.G. Nahas, ed. Marihuana:
       Chemistry, Biochemistry, and Cellular Effects. New York:
       Springer-Verlag, pp. 223-241.

826. JAKUBOVIC, A., and MC GEER, P.L. (1977) 'Biochemical changes
       in rat testicular cells in vitro produced by cannabinoids
       and alcohol: Metabolism and incorporation of labeled glu-
       cose, amino acids, and nucleic acid precursors.' Tox-
       icology and Applied Pharmacology, 41, 473-486.

827. JAKUBOVIC, A., MC GEER, E.G., and MC GEER, P.L. (1979) 'Ef-
       fects of cannabinoids on testosterone and protein systhesis
       in rat testis Leydig cells in vitro.' Molecular Cellular
       Endocrinology, 15, 41-50.

828. JAKUBOVIC, A., MC GEER, E.G., and MC GEER, P.L. (1980) 'Bio-
       chemical alterations induced by cannabinoids in the Leydig
       cells of the rat testis in vitro: Effects on testosterone
       and protein synthesis.' In: G.G. Nahas and W.D.M. Paton,
       eds. Marihuana: Biological Effects. Oxford: Pergamon
       Press, pp. 251-264.

829. JOHNSTON, W.C. (1968) 'A descriptive study of 100 convicted
       female narcotic residents.' Journal of Corrective Psy-
       chiatric and Social Thinking, 14, 230-236.

830. KAYMAKCALAN, S., ERCAN, Z.S., and TÜRKER, R.K. (1975) 'The
        evidence of the release of prostaglandin-like material
        from rabbit kidney and guinea-pig lung by (-)-trans-
        delta-9-tetrahydrocannabinol.' Journal of Pharmacy and
        Pharmacology, 27, 564-568.

831. KOFF, W.C. (1974) 'Marihuana and sexual activity.' Journal
        of Sexual Research, 10, 194- 200.

832. KOLODNY, R.C. (1975) 'Research issues in the study of mari-
        juana and male reproductive physiology in humans.' In:
        Marijuana and Health Hazards (Methodological Issues in
        Current Research). New York: Academic Press, pp. 71-81.

833. KOLODNY, R.C., LESSIN, P., TORO, G., MASTERS, W.H., and COHEN,
        J. (1976) 'Depression of plasma testosterone with acute
        marihuana administration.' In: M.C. Braude and S. Szara,
        eds. Pharmacology of Marihuana. New York: Raven Press,
        pp. 217-223.

834. KOLODNY, R.C., MASTERS, W.H., KOLODNER, R.M., and TORO, G.
        (1974) 'Depresssion of plasma testosterone levels after
        chronic intensive marihuana use.' New England Journal of
        Medicine, 290, 872-374.

835. KOLODNY, R.C., WEBSTER, S.K., TULLMAN, G.D., and DORNBUSH, R.I.
        (1979) 'Chronic marihuana use by women: Menstrual cycle
        and endocrine findings.' Presented at New York University
        Postgraduate Medical School Second Annual Conference on
        Marihuana: Marihuana--Biomedical Effects and Social Impli-
        cations, June 28-29.

836. KRAMER, J., and BEN-DAVID, M. (1974) 'Suppression of prolactin
        secretion by acute administration of delta-9-tetrahydro-
        cannabinol in rats.' Proceedings of the Society for
        Experimental Biology and Medicine, 147, 482-484.

837. LARES, A., OCHOA, Y., BOLAÑOS, A., APONTE, N., and MONTENEGRO, M.
        (1981) 'Effects of the resin and smoke condensate of
        Cannabis sativa on the oestrous cycle of the rat.' Bul-
        letin on Narcotics, 33, 55-61.

838. LEMBERGER, L., CRABTREE, R., ROWE, H., and CLEMENS, J. (1973)
        'Tetrahydrocannabinols and serum prolactin levels in man.'
        Life Sciences, 16, 1339-1343.

839. LEWIS, B. (1970) The Sexual Power of Marijuana. New York:
        Peter H. Wyden.

840. LING, G.M., THOMAS, J.A., USHER, D.R., and SINGHAL, R.L. (1973)
        'Effects of chronically administered delta-1-tetrahydro-
        cannabinol on adrenal and gonadal activity of male rats.'
        International Journal of Clinical Pharmacology, Therapy,
        and Toxicology, 7, 1-5.

841. LIST, A., NAZAR, B., NYQUIST, S., and HARCLERODE, J. (1977)
     'The effects of delta-9-tetrahydrocannabinol and cannabidiol
     on the metabolism of gonadal steroids in the rat.' Drug
     Metabolism and Disposition, 5, 268-272.

842. MARKS, B.H. (1973) 'Delta-1-tetrahydrocannabinol and lutein-
     izing hormone secretion.' Progress in Brain Research, 39,
     331-338.

843. MASKARINEC, M.P., SHIPLEY, G., NOVOTNY, M., BROWN, D.J., and
     FORNEY, R.B. (1978) 'Different effects of synthetic
     delta-9-tetrahydrocannabinol and cannabis extract on
     steroid metabolism in male rats.' Experientia, 34, 88-89.

844. MAUGH, T.H. (1975) 'Marihuana: New support for immune and
     reproductive hazards.' Science, 190, 865-867.

845. MC LEAN, B.K., RUBEL, A., and NIKITOVITCH-WINER, M.B. (1977)
     'Diurnal variation of follicle stimulating hormone (FSH)
     in the male rat.' Neuroendocrinology, 23, 23-30.

846. MENDELSON, J.H. (1976) 'Brief guide to office counseling:
     Marihuana and sex.' Medical Aspects of Human Sexuality,
     10, 23-24.

847. MENDELSON, J.H. (1981) 'Marijuana and sex.' Medical Aspects
     of Human Sexuality, 15, 141-152.

848. MENDELSON, J.H., ELLINGBOE, J., KUEHNLE, J.C., and MELLO, N.K.
     (1978) 'Effects of chronic marihuana use on integrated
     plasma testosterone and luteinizing hormone levels.'
     Journal of Pharmacology and Experimental Therapeutics, 207,
     611-617.

849. MENDELSON, J.H., KUEHNLE, J., ELLINGBOE, J., and BABOR, T.F.
     (1974) 'Plasma testosterone levels before, during, and
     after chronic marihuana smoking.' New England Journal
     of Medicine, 291, 1051-1055.

850. MENDELSON, J.H., KUEHNLE, J., ELLINGBOE, J., and BABOR, T.F.
     (1975) 'Effects of maijuana on plasma testosterone.'
     In: Marijuana and Health Hazards: Methodological Issues
     in Current Research. New York: Academic Press, Chapter 10,
     pp. 83-93.

851. MERARI, A., BARAK, A., and PLAVES, M. (1973) 'Effects of delta-
     1(2)-tetrahydrocannabinol on copulation in the male rat.'
     Psychopharmacologia, 28, 243-246.

852. MULINAS, M.G., and POMERANTZ, L. (1941) 'Pituitary replacement
     therapy in pseudohypophysectomy.' Endocrinology, 29,
     558-566.

853. NAHAS, G.G. (1977) 'Biomedical aspects of cannabis usage.'
     Bulletin on Narcotics, 29, 13-27.

854. NAHAS, G.G.   (1981) 'Brief guide to office counseling: Mari-
        juana and sex.' Medical Aspects of Human Sexuality, 15,
        30, 39.

855. NATIONAL COMMISSION ON MARIHUANA AND DRUG ABUSE.   (1972) 'Mari-
        huana and sexual behavior.' In: Marihuana: A Signal of
        Misunderstanding. Volume 1. Washington, D.C.: U.S. Gov-
        ernment Printing Office, Appendix, pp. 434-439.

856. NICOLAU, M., LAPA, A.J., and VALLE, J.R.   (1978) 'The inhibitory
        effects induced by delta-9-tetrahydrocannabinol on the con-
        tractions of the isolated rat vas deferens.' Archives
        Internationales de Pharmacodynamie et de Therapie, 236, 131-
        136.

857. NIR, I., AYALON, D., TSAFRIRI, A., CORDOVA, T., and LINDNER, H.R.
        (1973) 'Suppression of the cyclic surge of luteinizing
        hormone secretion and of ovulation in the rat by delta-1-
        tetrahydrocannabinol.' Nature, 243, 470-4 .

858. NOWLIS, V.   (1975) 'Categories of interest in the scientific
        search for relationships (i.e., interactions, associations,
        comparisons).' In: M. Sandler and D.L. Gessa, eds.
        Sexual Behavior: Pharmacology and Biochemistry. New York:
        Raven Press.

859. OKEY, A.B., and BONDY, G.P.   (1977) 'Is delta-9-tetrahydro-
        cannabinol estrogenic?' Science, 195, 904-905.

860. OKEY, A.B., and BONDY, G.P.   (1978) 'Delta-9-tetrahydrocannabin-
        ol and 17-beta-estradiol bind to different macromolecules
        in estrogen target tissues.' Science, 200, 312-315.

861. OKEY, A.B., and TRUANT, G.S.   (1975) 'Cannabis demasculinizes
        rats but is not estrogenic.' Life Sciences, 17, 1113-1117.

862. PARK, Y.Y., and TILTON, B.E.   (1970) 'Effects of marihuana
        smoke on avoidance response in rats.' Proceedings of the
        Western Pharmacology Society, 13, 151-155.

863. PUDER, M., NIR, D., AYALON, D., CORDOVA, T., and LINDNER, H.R.
        (1980) 'Effect of THC on basal and PGE_2 or Gn-RH-induced
        LH release in female rats.' Research Communications in
        Substance Abuse, 1, 407-426.

864. PUROHIT, V., AHLUWAHLIA, B.S., and VIGERSKY, R.A.   (1980)
        'Marihuana inhibits dihydrotestosterone binding to the
        androgen receptor.' Endocrinology, 107, 848-850.

865. PUROHIT, V., SINGH, H., and AHLUWALIA, B.S.   (1979) 'Evidence
        that the effects of methadone and marihuana on male repro-
        ductive organs are mediated at different sites on rats.'
        Biology of Reproduction, 20, 1039-1044.

866. RAINE, J.M., WING, D.R., and PATON, W.D.M. (1978) 'The effects
      of delta-1-tetrahydrocannabinol on mammary gland growth,
      enzyme activity, and plasma prolactin levels in the mouse.'
      European Journal of Pharmacology, 51, 11-17.

867. RAWITCH, A.B., SHULTZ, G.S., EBNER, K.E., and VARDARIS, R.M.
      (1977) 'Competition of delta-9-tetrahydrocannabinol with
      estrogen in rat uterine estrogen receptor binding.' Sci-
      ence, 197, 1189-1192.

868. ROCKWELL, K., ELLINWOOD, E., KANTON, C., MAACK, W., and
      SCHRUMPF, J. (1973) 'Drugs and sex: Scene of ambival-
      ence.' Journal of the American College and Health Assoc-
      iation, 21, 483-488.

869. ROSE, R.M. (1975) 'Background paper on testosterone and
      marijuana.' In: J.R. Tinklenberg, ed. Marihuana and
      Health Hazards: Methodological Issues in Current Re-
      search. New York: Academic Press, pp. 63-69.

870. ROSENKRANTZ, H., and HAYDEN, D.W. (1979) 'Acute and subacute
      inhalation toxicity of Turkish marihuana, cannabichromene,
      and cannabidiol in rats.' Toxicology and Applied Pharm-
      acology, 48, 375-386.

871. ROSENKRANTZ, H., HEYMAN, I.A., and BRAUDE, M.C. (1974) 'Inha-
      lation, parenteral and oral LD$_{50}$ values of delta-9-tetra-
      hydrocannabinol in Fischer rats.' Toxicology and Applied
      Pharmacology, 28, 18- .

872. ROSENKRANTZ, H., SPRAGUE, R.A., FLEISCHMAN, R.W., and BRUADE,
      M.C. (1975) 'Oral delta-9-tetrahydrocannabinol toxicity
      in rats treated for periods up to six months.' Toxicology
      and Applied Pharmacology, 32, 399-406.

873. RUBIN, V., and COMITAS, L. (1976) Ganja in Jamaica. New York:
      Anchor Books.

874. SASSENRATH, E.N., and CHAPMAN, L.F. (1975) 'Tetrahydrocanna-
      binol-induced manifestations of the "marihuana syndrome"
      in group-living macaques.' Federation Proceedings, 34,
      1666-16 .

875. SCHAEFER, C.F., GUNN, C.G., and DUBOWSKI, K.M. (1975) 'Normal
      plasma testosterone concentrations after marihuana smoking.'
      New England Journal of Medicine, 292, 867-868.

876. SCHWARZ, S., HARCLERODE, J., and NYQUIST, S.E. (1978) 'Effects
      of delta-9-tetrahydrocannabinol administration on marker
      proteins of rat testicular cells.' Life Sciences, 22, 7-14.

877. SHAHAR, A., and BINO, T. (1974) 'In vitro effects of delta-9-
      tetrahydrocannabinol (THC) on bull sperm.' Biochemical
      Pharmacology, 23, 1341-1342.

878. SHOEMAKER, R.H., and HARMON, J.W.   (1977) 'Suggested mechanism
      for demasculinizing effects of marihuana.' Federation
      Proceedings, 36, 345

879. SIEBER, B., FRISCHKNECHT, H.-R., and WASER, P.G.   (1980)
      'Behavioral effects of hashish in mice. I. Social inter-
      actions and nest-building behavior of males.' Psycho-
      pharmacology, 70, 149-154.

880. SMITH, C.G., BESCH, N.F., and ASCH, R.H.   (1980) 'Effects of
      marihuana on the reproductive system.' In: J.A. Thomas
      and R. Singhal, eds. Advances in Sex Hormone Research.
      Volume 4. Baltimore, Maryland: Urbin-Schwartzenberg,
      pp. 273-294.

881. SMITH, C.G., BESCH, N.F., SMITH, R.G., and BESCH, P.K.   (1979)
      'Effect of tetrahydrocannabinol on the hypothalamic-
      pituitary axis in the ovariectomized rhesus monkey.'
      Fertility and Sterility, 31, 335-341.

882. SMITH, C.G., SMITH, M.T., BESCH, N.F., SMITH, R.G., and ASCH,
      R.H. (1980) 'Effect of delta-9-tetrahydrocannabinol (THC)
      on female reproductive function.' In: G.G. Nahas and
      W.D.M. Paton, eds. Marihuana: Biological Effects. Oxford:
      Pergamon Press, pp. 449-456.

883. SOLOMON, J., COCCHIA, R., GRAY, D., SHATTUCK, D., and VOSSMER, A.
      (1976) 'Uterotrophic effect of delta-9-tetrahydrocannabinol
      in ovariectomized rats.' Science, 192, 559-561.

884. SPRONCK, H.J.W., LUTEIJN, J.M., SALEMINK, C.A., and NUGTEREN, D.H.
      (1978) 'Inhibition of prostaglandin biosynthesis by deriv-
      atives of olivetol formed under pyrolysis of cannabidiol.'
      Biochemical Pharmacology, 27, 607-608.

885. SYMONS, A.M., TEALE, J.D., and MARKS, V.   (1976) 'Effect of
      delta-9-tetrahydrocannabinol on the hypothalamic-pituitary-
      gonadal system in the maturing male rat.' Journal of
      Endocrinology, 67, 43P-44P.

886. TART, C.T. (1971) On Being Stoned. Palo Alto, California:
      Science and Behavior Books.

887. THOMPSON, G.R., FLEISHMAN, R.W., ROSENKRANTZ, H., and BRAUDE,
      M.C. (1974) 'Oral and intravenous toxicity of delta-9-
      tetrahydrocannabinol in rhesus monkeys.' Toxicology and
      Applied Pharmacology, 27, 648-654.

888. THOMPSON, G.R., MASON, M.M., ROSENKRANTZ, H., and BRAUDE, M.C.
      (1973) 'Chronic oral toxicity of cannabinoids in rats.'
      Toxicology and Applied Pharmacology, 25, 373-379.

889. TURLEY, W.A., and FLOODY, O.R. (1981) 'Delta-9-tetrahydrocannabinol stimulates receptive and proceptive sexual behaviors in female hamsters.' Pharmacology, Biochemistry, and Behavior, 14, 745-747.

890. TURNER, J.C., HEMPHILL, J.K., and MAHLBERG, P.G. (1981) 'Interrelationships of glandular trichomes and cannabinoid content. II. Developing vegetative leaves of Cannabis sativa L. (Cannabaceae).' Bulletin on Narcotics, 33, 63-71.

891. TYREY, L. (1978) 'Delta-9-tetrahydrocannabinol suppression of episodic luteinizing hormone secretion in the ovariectomized rat.' Endocrinology, 102, 1808.

892. TYREY, L. (1980) 'Delta-9-tetrahydrocannabinol: A potent inhibitor of episodic luteinizing hormone secretion.' Journal of Pharmacology and Experimental Therapeutics, 213, 306-308.

893. UYENO, E.T. (1976) 'Effects of delta-9-tetrahydrocannabinol and 2,5-dimethoxy-4-methylamphetamine on rat sexual dominance behavior.' Proceedings of the Western Pharmacology Society, 19, 369-372.

894. VIRGO, B.B. (1979) 'The estrogenicity of delta-9-tetrahydrocannabinol (THC): THC neither blocks nor induces ovum implantation, nor does it effect uterine growth.' Research Communications in Chemistry, Pathology, and Pharmacology, 25, 65.

895. VYAS, D.K., and SINGH, R. (1976) 'Effect of cannabis and opium on the testis of the pigeon Columba livia Gmelin.' Indian Journal of Experimental Biology, 14, 22-25.

896. WADDELL, T.G., JONES, H., and KEITH, A.L. (1980) 'Legendary chemical aphrodisiacs.' Journal of Chemical Education, 57, 341-342.

897. WEINER, R., and STILLMAN, D. (1979) Woodstock Census: The Nationwide Survey of the Sixties Generation. New York: Viking Press.

898. WILSON, E. (1949) 'Crazy dreamers.' Collier's, 123, 27.

899. ZIMMERMAN, A.M., BRUCE, W.R., and ZIMMERMAN, S. (1979) 'Effects of cannabinoids on sperm morphology.' Pharmacology, 18, 143-148.

900. ZIMMERMAN, A.M., ZIMMERMAN, S., and RAJ, A.Y. (1980) 'Effects of cannabinoids on spermatogenesis in mice.' In: G.G. Nahas and W.D.P. Paton, eds. Marihuana: Biological Effects. Oxford: Pergamon Press, p. 407.

901.   ZINBERG, N.E.   (1974)   'Marijuana and sex.'   [Letter.]
       New England Journal of Medicine, 291, 309-310.

902.   ZUCKERMAN, M., BONE, R., NEARY, A., MANGELSDORFF, D., and
       BRUSTMAN, B.   (1972)   'What is the sensation seeker?
       Personality trait and experience correlates of the
       sensation-seeking scales.'   Journal of Consulting and
       Clinical Psychology, 39, 308-321.

Methaqualone

903. FALCO, M. (1976) 'Methaqualone misuse: Foreign experience and United States drug control policy.' International Journal of the Addictions, 11, 597-610.

904. GERALD, M.C., and SCHWIRIAN, P.M. (1973) 'Nonmedical use of methaqualone.' Archives of General Psychiatry, 28, 627-631.

905. HOLLISTER, L.E. (1975) 'Drugs and sexual behavior in man.' Life Sciences, 17, 661-667.

906. INABA, D.S., GAY, G.R., NEWMAYER, J.A., and WHITEHEAD, C. (1973) 'Methaqualone abuse: "Luding out."' Journal of the American Medical Association, 224, 1505-1509.

907. KOCHANSKY, G.E., HEMENWAY, T., SALZMAN, C., and SHADER, R. (1975) 'Methaqualone abusers: A preliminary survey of college students.' Diseases of the Nervous System, 36, 348-351.

908. KRAMER, S. (1973) 'Methaqualone as aphrodisiac.' American Journal of Psychiatry, 130, 1044.

909. WEISSBERG, K. (1972) 'Sopers are a bummer.' Berkeley Barb, Sept. 1-7, 13.

Narcotics

910. ADAMS, J.W. (1978) *Psychoanalysis of Drug Dependence*. New York: Grune and Stratton.

911. AZIZI, F., VAGENAKIS, A.G., LONGCOPE, C., INGBAR, S.H., and BRAVERMAN, L.E. (1973) 'Decreased serum testosterone concentration in male heroin and methadone addicts.' *Steroids*, 22, 467-472.

912. BAHNA, G., and GORDON, N.B. (1978) 'Rehabilitation experiences of women ex-addicts in methadone treatment.' *International Journal of the Addictions*, 13, 639-655.

913. BAI, J., GREENWALD, E., CATERINE, H., and KAMINETZKY, H. (1974) 'Drug-related menstrual aberrations.' *Obstetrics and Gynecology*, 44, 713-719.

914. BARRACLOUGH, C.A., and SAWYER, C.H. (1955) 'Inhibition of the release of pituitary ovulatory hormone in the rat by morphine.' *Endocrinology*, 57, 329-337.

915. BECKETT, H.D., and LODGE, K.J. (1971) 'Aspects of social relationships in human addicts admitted for treatment.' *Bulletin on Narcotics*, 23, 29-36.

916. BERZINS, J., ROSS, W., and MONROE, J. (1971) 'A multivariate study of the personality characteristics of hospitalised narcotic addicts on the M.M.P.L.' *Journal of Clinical Psychology*, 27, 174-181.

917. BLATMAN, S. (1971) 'Neonatal and followup.' In: United States Department of Health, Education, and Welfare. *Proceedings of the Third National Conference on Methandone Treatment, November 14-16, 1970*. Washington, D.C.: U.S. Government Printing Office; Rockville, Maryland: Public Health Service Publication No. 2172, pp. 82-85.

918. BLINICK, G. (1968) 'Menstrual function and pregnancy in narcotics addicts treated with methadone.' *Nature*, 219, 180.

919. BLINICK, G. (1971) 'Fertility of narcotics addicts and effects
      of addiction in the offspring.' Social Biology, 18, S34-S39.

920. BLINICK, G. (1971) 'Obstetrical aspects through the delivery
      room.' In: United States Department of Health, Education,
      and Welfare. Proceedings of the Third National Conference
      on Methadone Treatment, November 14-16, 1970. Washington,
      D.C.: U.S. Government Printing Office; Rockville, Maryland:
      Public Health Service Publication No. 2172, pp. 80-82.

921. BLINICK, G., JEREZ, E., and WALLACH, R.C. (1977) 'Pregnancy and
      drug abuse.' In: S.N. Pradhan and S.N. Dutta, eds. Drug
      Abuse: Clinical and Basic Aspects. St. Louis, Missouri:
      C.V. Mosby.

922. BLINICK, G., WALLACH, R.C., and JEREZ, E. (1972) 'Methadone and
      pregnancy.' In: A. Goldstein, ed. Fourth National Con-
      ference on Methadone Treatment. New York: National Assoc-
      iation for the Prevention of Addiction to Narcotics, pp. 129-
      131.

923. BLOCH, I. (1933) Anthropological Studies in the Strange Sexual
      Practices of All Races in All Ages, Ancient and Modern.
      New York: Anthropological Press.

924. BLOOM, W.A., JR., and BUTCHER, B.T. (1971) 'Methadone side
      effects and related symptoms in 200 methadone maintenance
      patients.' In: United States Department of Health, Edu-
      cation, and Welfare. Proceedings of the Third National Con-
      ference on Methadone Treatment, November 14-16, 1970.
      Washington, D.C.: U.S. Government Printing Office; Rock-
      ville, Maryland: Public Health Service Publication No. 2172,
      pp. 44-47.

925. BOLELLI, G., LAFISCA, S., FLAMIGNI, C., LODI, S., FRANCES-
      CHETTI, F., FILICORI, M., and MOSCA, R. (1979) 'Heroin
      addiction: Relationship between the plasma levels of testos-
      terone, dyhydrotestosterone, androstenedione, LH, FSH, and
      the plasma concentration of heroin.' Toxicology, 15, 19-29.

926. BOWDEN, C. (1971) 'Determinants of initial use of opioids.'
      Comprehensive Psychiatry, 12, 136-140.

927. BRAMBILLA, F., SACCHETTI, E., and BRUNETTA, M. (1977)
      'Pituitary-gonadal function in heroin addicts.' Neuro-
      psychobiology, 3, 160-166.

928. BRUNI, J.F., VAN VUGT, D., MARSHALL, S., and MEITES, J. (1977)
      'Effects of naloxone, morphine, and methionine enkephalin
      on serum prolactin, luteinizing hormone, follicle stim-
      ulating hormone, thyroid stimulating hormone, and growth
      hormone.' Life Sciences, 21, 461-466.

929. BRUNC, F., and FERRACUTI, F. (1977) 'Drugs and sexual behavior.'
      Quoderni di Criminologia Clinica, 19, 17-36.

930. BUCKMAN, J.   (1971)   'Psychology of drug abuse.'   Medical College
      of Virginia Quarterly, 7, 98-102.

931. BUCKY, S.F.   (1973)   'The relationship between background and ex-
      tent of heroin use.'   American Journal of Psychiatry, 130,
      709-710.

932. BURROUGHS, W.   (1953)   Junkie.   New York: Ace Books.

933. CASSIDY, W.J.   (1972)   'Maintenance methadone treatment of drug
      dependency.'   Journal of the Canadian Psychiatric Assoc-
      iation, 17, 107-115.

934. CHAMBERS, C.D., BRILL, L., and LANGROD, J.   (1973)   'Physio-
      logical and psychological side effects reported during
      maintenance therapy.   In: C.D. Chambers and L. Brill, eds.
      Methadone: Experiences and Issues.   New York: Behavioral
      Publications, pp. 163-170.

935. CHEIN, I., GERARD, D.L., LEE, R.S., and ROSENFELD, E.   (1964)
      The Road to H.   New York: Basic Books.

936. CHESSICK, R.   (1960)   'The "pharmacogenic orgasm" in the drug
      addict.'   Archives of General Psychiatry, 3, 545-556.

937. CHOPRA, R.N., and CHOPRA, I.C.   (1955)   'Quasi-medical use of
      opium in India and its effects.'   Bulletin on Narcotics,
      7, 1.

938. CICERO, T.J.   (1977)   'An in vivo assay for the analysis of the
      biological potency and structure-activity relationships of
      narcotics: Serum testosterone depletion in the male rat.'
      Journal of Pharmacology and Experimental Therapeutics, 202,
      670-675.

939. CICERO, T.J.   (1980)   'Effects of exogenous and endogenous
      opiates on the hypothalamic-pituitary-gonanal axis in the
      male.'   Federation Proceedings, 39, 2551-2554.

940. CICERO, T.J., BADGER, T.M., WILCOX, C.E., BELL, R.D., and
      MEYER, E.R.   (1977)   'Morphine decreases luteinizing hormone
      by an action on the hypothalamic-pituitary axis.'   Journal
      of Pharmacology and Experimental Therapeutics, 203, 548,
      555.

941. CICERO, T.J., BELL, R.D., MEYER, E.R., and SCHWEITZER, J.   (1976)
      'Narcotics and the hypothalamic-pituitary-gonadal axis:
      Acute effects on luteinizing hormone, testosterone, and
      androgen dependent systems.'   Journal of Pharmacology and
      Experimental Therapeutics, 201, 76-83.

942. CICERO, T.J., BELL, R.D., WIEST, W.G., ALLISON, J.H., POLA-
      KOSKI, K., and ROBINS, E.   (1975)   'Function of the male
      sex organs in heroin and methadone users.'   New England
      Journal of Medicine, 292, 882-887.

943. CICERO, T.J., MEYER, E.R., BELL, R.D., and KOCH, G.A. (1976)
      'Effects of morphine and methadone on testosterone,
      luteinizing hormone and the secondary sex organs of the
      male rat.' Endocrinology, 98, 365-370.

944. CICERO, T.J., MEYER, E.R., BELL, R.D., and WIEST, W. (1974)
      'Effects of morphine on the secondary sex organs and plasma
      testosterone levels of rats.' Research Communications in
      Chemistry, Pathology, and Pharmacology, 7, 17-24.

945. CICERO, T.J., MEYER, E.R., GABRIEL, S.M., BELL, R.D., and WIL-
      COX, C.E. (1980) 'Morphine exerts testosterone-like ef-
      fects in the hypothalamus of the castrated male rat.' Brain
      Research, 202, 151-164.

946. CICERO, T.J., MEYER, E.R., GABRIEL, S.M., and WILCOX, C.E. (1980)
      'Androgenic-like effects of morphine in the male rat.'
      National Institute of Drug Abuse Research Monograph Series,
      34, 152-158.

947. CICERO, T.J., MEYER, E.R., WIEST, W.G., OLNEY, J.W., and BELL,
      R.D. (1975) 'Effects of chronic morphine administration
      on the reproductive system of the male rat.' Journal of
      Pharmacology and Experimental Therapeutics, 192, 542-548.

948. CICERO, T.J., SCHAINKER, B.A., and MEYER, E.R. (1979) 'Endogen-
      ous opioids participate in the regulation of the hypothal-
      amic-pituitary-luteinizing hormone and testosterone's
      negative feedback control of luteinizing hormone.' Endo-
      crinology, 104, 1286-1291.

949. CICERO, T.J., WILCOX, C.E., BELL, R.D., and MEYER, E.R. (1976)
      'Acute reductions in serum testosterone levels by narcotics
      in the male rat: Stereospecificity, blockade by naloxone
      and tolerance.' Journal of Pharmacology and Experimental
      Therapeutics, 198, 340-346.

950. CLARK, J., CAPEL, W., GOLDSMITH, B., and STEWART, G. (1972)
      'Marriage and methadone: Spouse behavior patterns in heroin
      addicts maintained on methadone.' Journal of Marriage and
      the Family, Vol.? 497-502.

951. COCTEAU, J. (1972) Opium: The Diary of a Cure. London: New
      English Library.

952. CROWLEY, T.J., HYDINGER, M., STYNES, A.J., and FEIGER, A. (1975)
      'Monkey motor stimulation and altered social behavior during
      chronic methadone administration.' Psychopharmacologica,
      43, 135-144.

953. CROWLEY, T.J., and SIMPSON, R. (1978) 'Methadone dose and human
      sexual behavior.' International Journal of the Addictions,
      13, 285-295.

954. CROWLEY, T.J., STYNES, A.J., HYDINGER, M., and KAUFMAN, I.C.
      (1974) 'Ethanol, methamphetamine, pentobarbital, morphine,
      and monkey social behavior.' Archives of General Psychiatry,
      31, 829-838.

955. CUSHMAN, P., JR. (1971) 'Some endocrinological aspects of
      heroin addiction and methadone maintenance therapy.' In:
      United States Department of Health, Education, and Welfare.
      Proceedings of the Third National Conference on Methadone
      Treatment, November 14-16, 1970. Washington, D.C.: U.S.
      Government Printing Office; Rockville, Maryland: Public
      Health Service Publication No. 2172, pp. 144-149.

956. CUSHMAN, P., JR. (1972) 'Sexual behavior in heroin addiction
      and methadone maintenance: Correlation with plasma lutein-
      izing hormone.' New York State Journal of Medicine, 72,
      1261-1265.

957. CUSHMAN, P., JR. (1973) 'Plasma testosterone in narcotic ad-
      diction.' American Journal of Medicine, 55, 452-458.

958. CUSHMAN, P., JR. (1980) 'The major medical sequelae of opioid
      addiction.' Drug and Alcohol Dependence, 5, 239-254.

959. CUSHMAN, P., JR., and DOLE, V. (1973) 'Detoxification of rehab-
      ilitated methadone maintenance patients.' Journal of the
      American Medical Association, 226, 747-752.

960. CUSHMAN, P., and KREEK, M.J. (1974) 'Methadone-maintained
      patients: Effect of methadone on plasma testosterone, FSH,
      LH, and prolactin.' New York State Journal of Medicine,
      74, 1970-1973.

961. CUSKEY, W.R., PREMKUMAR, T., and SIGEL, L. (1972) 'Survey of
      opiate addiction among females in the U.S. between 1850 and
      1970.' Public Health Review, 1, 6.

962. DE LEON, G., and WEXLER, H. (1973) 'Heroin addiction: Its re-
      lation to sexual behavior and sexual experience.' Journal
      of Abnormal Psychology, 81, 36-38.

963. DENSEN-GERBER, J. (1972) 'Sexual behavior, abortion, and birth
      control in heroin addicts: Legal and psychiatric consider-
      ations.' Contemporary Drug Problems, 1, 783-793.

964. DENSEN-GERBER, J., WIENER, M., and HOCHSTEDLER, N. (1972)
      'Sexual behavior, abortion, and birth control in human ad-
      dicts: Legal and psychiatric considerations.' Contemporary
      Drug Problems, 1, 783-793.

965. DING, L.K. (1972) 'The role of sex in narcotic addiction in
      Hong Kong.' Asian Journal of Medicine, 8, 119-121.

966. DOBRIN, E.I., and MARES, S.E. (1974) 'Effects of morphine on
      serum gonadotropin levels.' In: M.J. Singh and H. Lal,
      eds. Drug Addiction. Volume 4: New Aspects of Analytical
      and Clinical Toxicology. New York: Stratton Intercontin-
      ental Medical Book Corp., pp. 69-77.

967. ELLINGBOE, J., MENDELSON, J.H., HOLBROOK, P.G., et al. (1978)
      'Maltrexone effects on luteinizing hormone (LH) secretion
      and mood states implicate endogenous opioid mechanism in
      regulation of the hypothalamic-pituitary-gonadal axis.'
      Federation Proceedings, 37, 275 (abstract).

968. ELLINWOOD, E.H., JR., SMITH, W.G., and VAILLANT, G.E. (1966)
      'Narcotic addiction in males and females: A comparison.'
      International Journal of the Addictions, 1, 33-45.

969. ESPEJO, R., HOGBEN, G., and STIMMEL, B. (1973) 'Sexual perfor-
      mance of men on methadone maintenance.' Proceedings of the
      National Conference of Methadone Treatment, 1, 490-493.

970. FEDERN, E.A. (1972) 'A psycho-social view of "drug-abuse" in
      adolescence.' Child Psychiatry and Human Development, 3,
      10-20.

971. FENICHEL, O. (1975) The Psychoanalytical Theory of Neurosis.
      New York: W.W. Norton.

972. FISHMAN, J., NORTON, B.I., and HAHN, E.F. (1980) 'Opiate reg-
      ulation of estradiol-2-hydroxylase in brains of male rats:
      Mechanism for control of pituitary hormone secretion.' Pro-
      ceedings of the National Academy of Sciences, 77, 2574-2576.

973. FORT, J.P. (1954) 'Heroin addiction among young men.' Psy-
      chiatry, 17, 251-259.

974. FREEDMAN, A. (1967) 'Drugs and sexual behavior.' Medical As-
      pects of Human Sexuality, 1, 25-31.

975. FREEDMAN, A. (1967) 'Psychopharmacological approaches to nar-
      cotic addiction.' In: H.Brill, J.Cole, P.Deniker, H.Hip-
      pius, and P.Bradley, eds. Neuropsychopharmacology.
      New York: Excerpta Medica.

976. GARBUTT, G., and GOLDSTEIN, A. (1972) 'Blind comparison of
      three methadone maintenance dosage in 180 patients.' In:
      Proceedings of the Fourth National Conference in Methadone
      Treatment. New York: National Association for Prevention
      of Addiction to Narcotics, pp. 411-415.

977. GARDNER, J. (1969) 'Indicators of homosexuality in the human
      figure drawings of heroin- and pill-using addicts.' Per-
      ceptual and Motor Skills, 28, 705-706.

978.   GAULDEN, E.C., LITTLEFIELD, D.C., PUTOFF, O.E., and SEIVERT, A.L.
       (1964) 'Menstrual abnormalities associated with heroin
       addiction.' American Journal of Obstetrics and Gynecology,
       90, 155-160.

979.   GEARING, F.R. (1971) 'Successes and failures in methadone main-
       tenance of heroin addiction in New York City.' In:
       United States Department of Health, Education, and Welfare.
       Proceedings of the Third National Conference on Methadone
       Treatment, November 14-16, 1970. Washington, D.C.: U.S.
       Government Printing Office; Rockville, Maryland: Public
       Health Service Publication No. 2172, pp. 2-16.

980.   GESSA, G., PAGLIETTI, E., and PELLIGRINI QUARANTOTH, B. (1979)
       'Induction of copulation between sexually inactive rats by
       naloxone.' Science, 204, 203-205.

981.   GLATT, M.M., et al. (1966) The Drug Scene in Great Britain:
       Journey to Loneliness. London: Arnold, p. 18.

982.   GLICK, B.B., BAUGHMAN, W.L., JENSEN, J.N., and PHOENIX, C.H.
       (1982) 'Endogenous opiate systems and primate reproduction:
       Inability of naloxone to induce sexual activity in Rhesus
       males.' Archives of Sexual Behavior, 11, 267-275.

983.   GOLDSTEIN, A. (1971) 'Blind controlled dosage comparisons with
       methadone in 200 patients.' In: United States Department
       of Health, Education, and Welfare. Proceedings of the Third
       National Conference on Methadone Treatment, November 14-16,
       1970. Washington, D.C.: U.S. Government Printing Office;
       Rockville, Maryland: Public Health Service Publication
       No. 2172, pp. 31-37.

984.   GOLDSTEIN, A. (1971) 'Blind dosage comparisons and other
       studies in a large methadone program.' Journal of Psych-
       edelic Drugs, 4, 177-181.

985.   GOLDSTEIN, A., and JUDSON, B.A. (1973) 'Efficacy and side ef-
       fects of 3 widely different methadone doses.' In: Pro-
       ceedings of the Fifth National Conference on Methadone
       Treatment. Washington, D.C.: U.S. Government Printing
       Office, pp. 21-44.

986.   HALL, M.E. (1932) 'Mental and physical efficiency of women
       drug addicts.' Journal of Abnormal and Social Psychology,
       33, 332-345.

987.   HANBURY, R., COHEN, M., and STIMMEL, B. (1977) 'Adequacy of
       sexual performance in men maintained on methadone.' Amer-
       ican Journal of Drug and Alcohol Abuse, 4, 13-20.

988.   HARGREAVES, W.A., LING, W., BROWN, T.C., WEINBERG, J.A., LANDS-
       BERG, R., and HARRISON, W.L. (1979) 'Women on LAAM main-
       tenance: Initial experiences.' Journal of Psychedelic
       Drugs, 11, 223-229.

989. HASTINGS, D.W. (1963) Impotence and Frigidity. Boston: Little, Brown, and Co.

990. HEMMINGS, R., FOX, G., and TOLIS, G. (1982) 'Effect of morphine on the hypothalamic-pituitary axis in postmenopausal women.' Fertility and Sterility, 37, 389-391.

991. HERTZ, R. (1971) 'Addiction, fertility, and pregnancy.' Social Biology, 18, S40-S41.

992. HETTA, J. (1977) 'Effects of morphine and naltrexone on sexual behavior of the male rat.' Acta Pharmacologica Toxicologica, 41 (Supplement 4), 53.

993. HOFFMAN, M. (1964) 'Drug addiction and "hypersexuality": Related modes of mastery.' Comprehensive Psychiatry, 5, 262-270.

994. IEIRI, T., CHEN, H.T., CAMPBELL, B.A., and MEITES, J. (1980) 'Effects of naloxone and morphine on the proestrous surge of prolactin and gonadotropins in the rat.' Endocrinology, 106, 1568-1570.

995. IEIRI, T., CHEN, H.T., and MEITES, J. (1979) 'Effects of morphine and naloxone on serum levels of luteinizing hormone and prolactin in prepubertal male and female rats.' Neuroendocrinology, 29, 288-292.

996. IEIRI, T., SUZUKI, H., and SHIMODA, S. (1980) 'Effects of naloxone and morphine on the proestrous surge of prolactin and gonadotropins in the rat.' [In Japanese.] Horumon-To-Rinsho, 28, 1017-1020.

997. IRWIN, J. (1975) 'The "normal" life of the addict and the consequences of addiction.' In: J. Irwin, ed. The Social Careers of Heroin Addicts. Washington, D.C.: National Institute on Drug Abuse, pp. 77-90.

998. JAKUBOVIC, A., and MC GEER, E.G. (1979) 'Narcotics and rat testicular metabolism.' Molecular Pharmacology, 16, 970-980.

999. JESSUP, M.A. (1979) 'Sexuality and illness. Heroin and methadone: Their impact on human sexuality.' MCN, 4, 367-370.

1000. JONES, H.D., and JONES, H.C. (1977) Sensual Drugs. New York: Cambridge University Press.

1001. JURGENSEN, W. (1966) 'Problems of inpatient treatment of addiction.' International Journal of the Addictions, 1, 62-73.

1002. KAUFMAN, E. (1974) 'The psychodynamics of opiate dependence: A new look.' American Journal of Drug and Alcohol Abuse, 1, 349-370.

1003. KRAFT, T. (1970) 'Drug addiction and personality disorder.' British Journal of Addiction, 64, 403-408.

1004. KRAUS, W.M. (1918) 'An analysis of the action of morphine upon the vegetative nervous system of man.' Journal of Nervous and Mental Diseases, 48, 269-273.

1005. KREEK, M.J. (1973) 'Medical safety and side effects of methadone in tolerant individuals.' Journal of the American Medical Association, 223, 665-668.

1006. KURLAND, A.A. (1978) Psychiatric Aspects of Opiate Dependence. West Palm Beach, Florida: CRC Press.

1007. KURTZBERG, R., CAVIOR, N., and LIPTON, D. (1966) 'Sex drawn first and sex drawn larger by opiate addict and non-addict inmates on the Draw-a-Person Test.' Journal of Protective Techniques, 30, 55-58.

1008. LA BELLA, F., HAVLICEK, V., PINSKY, C., and LEYBIN, L. (1978) 'Opiate-like naloxone-reversible effects on androsterone sulfate in rats.' Canadian Journal of Physiological Pharmacology, 56, 940-944.

1009. LAFISCA, S., BOLELLI, G., FRANCESCHETTI, F., FILICORI, M., FLAMIGNY, C., and MARISO, M. (1981) 'Hormone levels in methadone-treated drug addicts.' Drug and Alcohol Dependence, 8, 229-234.

1110. LANDEN, B., and LANDEN, N. (1967) 'A cross-cultural study of narcotic addiction in New York.' In: Vocational Rehabilitation Advances in Rehabilitating the Narcotic Addict. Washington, D.C.: U.S. Government Printing Office, pp. 359-369.

1111. LANGROD, J., LOWINSON, J., and RUIZ, P. (1981) 'Methadone treatment and physical complaints: A clinical analysis.' International Journal of the Addictions, 16, 947-952.

1112. LASKOWITZ, D. (1964) 'Psychological characteristics of the adolescent addict.' In: E. Harms, ed. Drug Addiction in Youth. New York: Pergamon Press.

1113. LA TENDRESSE, J.D. (1968) 'Masturbation and its relation to addiction.' Review of Existential Psychology and Psychiatry, 8, 16-17.

1114. LAURIE, P. (1967) Drugs. New York: Penguin Books.

1115. LEHTINEN, A.M. (1981) 'Opiate action on adenohypophyseal hormone secretion during anesthesia and gynecologic surgery in different phases of the menstrual cycle.' Acta Anaesthesiologica Scandinavica (Supplement), 25, 1-54.

1116. LICHTENSTEIN, P.M. (1914) 'Narcotic addiction.' New York Medical Journal, 100, 962-966.

1117. LINKEN, A. (1968) 'A study of drug-taking among young patients
       attending a clinic for venereal disease.' British Journal
       of Venereal Diseases, 44, 337-341.

1118. LINTERN-MOORE, S., SUPASRI, Y., PAVASUTHIPAISIT, K., and SOBHON, P.
       (1979) 'Acute and chronic morphine sulfate treatment alters
       ovarian development in prepuberal rats.' Biology and Repro-
       duction, 21, 379-383.

1119. LONGWELL, B., KESTLER, R.J., and COX, T.J. (1979) 'Side effects
       in methadone patients: A survey of self-reported com-
       plaints.' International Journal of the Addictions, 14,
       485-494.

1120. MAGID, M.O. (1929) 'Narcotic drug addiction in the female.'
       Medical Journal and Record, 129, 306-310.

1121. MARTIN, C.A., and MARTIN, W.R. (1980) 'Opiate dependence in
       women.' In: O.R. Kalant, ed. Alcohol and Drug Problems
       in Women. New York: Plenum Publishing Company, pp. 465-
       485.

1122. MARTIN, W.R., HEWETT, B.B., BAKER, A.J., and HAERTZEN, C.A.
       (1977) 'Aspects of the psychopathology and pathophysiology
       of addiction.' Drug and Alcohol Dependence, 2, 185-202.

1123. MARTIN, W.R., JASINSKI, D.R., HAERTZEN, C.A., KAY, P.C., JONES,
       B.E., MANSKY, P.A., and CARPENTER, R.W. (1973) 'Methadone--
       a reevaluation.' Archives of General Psychiatry, 28, 286-295.

1124. MASLANSKY, R.A., SUKOV, R., and BEAUMONT, G. (1971) 'Pregnan-
       cies in methadone maintained mothers: A preliminary report.'
       In: United States Department of Health, Education, and
       Welfare. Proceedings of the Third National Conference on
       Methadone Treatment, November 14-16, 1970. Washington, D.C.:
       U.S. Government Printing Office; Rockville, Maryland: Pub-
       lic Health Service Publication No. 2172, pp. 56-61.

1125. MASTENS, R.E.L. (1962) Forbidden Sexual Behavior and Morality.
       New York: Julian Press.

1126. MATHES, J.L. (1970) 'Sexual aspects of human addiction.' Med-
       ical Aspects of Human Sexuality, 4, 98-109.

1127. MC INTOSH, T.K., VALLANO, M.L., and BARFIELD, R.J. (1980) 'Ef-
       fects of morphine, beta-endorphin and naloxone on catechol-
       amine levels and sexual behavior in the male rat.' Pharma-
       cology, Biochemistry, and Behavior, 13, 435-441.

1128. MC NAMEE, H.B. (1980) 'Opiate use and sexual function in women.'
       [Letter.] American Journal of Psychiatry, 137, 1628.

1129. MENDELSON, J.H., ELLINGBOE, J., KUEHNLE, J.C., and MELLO, N.K. (1978) 'Effect of chronic marihuana use on integrated plasma testosterone and luteinizing hormone levels.' Journal of Pharmacology and Experimental Therapeutics, 207, 661-671.

1130. MENDELSON, J.H., ELLINGBOE, J., KUEHNLE, J.C., and MELLO, N.K. (1979) 'Effect of naltrexone on mood and neuroendocrine function in normal adult males.' Psychoneuroendocrinology, 3, 231-236.

1131. MENDELSON, J.H., ELLINGBOE, J., KUEHNLE, J.C., and MELLO, N.K. (1979) 'Heroin and naltrexone effects on pituitary-gonadal hormones in man: Tolerance and supersensitivity.' National Institute of Drug Abuse Research Monograph Series, 27, 302-308.

1132. MENDELSON, J.H., ELLINGBOE, J., KUEHNLE, J.C., and MELLO, N.K. (1980) 'Heroin and naltrexone effects on pituitary-gonadal hormones in man: Interaction of steroid feedback effects, tolerance, and supersensitivity.' Journal of Pharmacology and Experimental Therapeutics, 214, 503-506.

1133. MENDELSON, J.H., and MELLO, N.K. (1975) 'Plasma tolerance levels during chronic heroin use and protracted abstinence, a study of Hong Kong addicts.' Clinical Pharmacology and Therapeutics, 17, 529-533.

1134. MENDELSON, J.H., MENDELSON, J.E., and PATCH, V.D. (1974) 'Effects of heroin and methadone on plasma testosterone in narcotic addicts.' Federation Proceedings, 33, 232.

1135. MENDELSON, J.H., MENDELSON, J.E., and PATCH, V.D. (1975) 'Plasma testosterone levels in heroin addiction and during methadone maintenance.' Journal of Pharmacology and Experimental Therapeutics, 192, 211-217.

1136. MENDELSON, J.H., MEYER, R.E., ELLINGBOE, J., MIRIN, S.M., and MC DOUGLE, M. (1975) 'Effects of heroin and methadone on plasma cortisol and testosterone.' Journal of Pharmacology and Experimental Therapeutics, 195, 296-302.

1137. MENNINGER-LERCHENTHAL, E. (1934) 'Schwangerschaft und Geburt morphinisticher Frauen.' ['Pregnancy and birth among morphine-addicted women.'] Zentralblatt Gynäk , 58, 1044.

1138. MEYERSON, B.J. (1981) 'Comparison of the effects of beta-endorphin and morphine on exploratory and socio-sexual behaviour in the male rat.' European Journal of Pharmacology, 69, 453-463.

1139. MILLS, L.C. (1975) 'Drug-induced impotence.' American Family Physician, 12, 104-106.

1140. MINTZ, J., O'HARE, K., O'BRIEN, C.P., and GOLDSCHMIDT, J. (1974)
       'Sexual problems of heroin addicts.' Archives of General
       Psychiatry, 31, 700-703.

1141. MIRIN, S.M., MENDELSON, J.H., ELLINGBOE, J., and MEYER, R.E.
       (1976) 'Acute effects of heroin and naltrexone on testos-
       terone and gonadotropin secretion: A pilot study.' Psycho-
       neuroendocrinology, 1, 359-369.

1142. MIRIN, S.M., MEYER, R.E., ELLINGBOE, J., and MENDELSON, J.H.
       (1979) 'Effects of opiates on neuroendocrine function:
       Testosterone and pituitary gonadotropins.' In: R.E. Meyer
       and S.M. Mirin, eds. The Human Stimulus: Implications for
       a Theory of Addiction. New York: Plenum Press, pp. 177-
       198.

1143. MIRIN, S.M., MEYER, R.E., MENDELSON, J.H., and ELLINGBOE, J.
       (1980) 'Opiate use and sexual function.' American Journal
       of Psychiatry, 137, 909-915.

1144. MORAT, D. (1911) 'Le sang et les secretions au cours de la
       morphinomanie et de la desintoxication.' [Blood and secretions
       in the course of morphine addiction and detoxification.']
       Thèse, Paris.

1145. MOTT, J. (1972) 'The psychological basis of drug addiction:
       The intellectual and personality characteristics of opiate
       users.' British Journal of Addiction, 67, 89-99.

1146. MURAKI, T., and TOKUNAGA, Y. (1977) 'Inhibitory effect of mor-
       phine on serum gonadotropins and prolactin of proestrous
       rats.' Journal of Pharmacology, 27, 461-462.

1147. MURAKI, T., TOKUNAGA, Y., and MAKINO, T. (1977) 'Effects of
       morphine and naloxone on serum LH, FSH, and prolactin levels
       and on hypothalamic content of LH-RF in proestrous rats.'
       [In Japanese.] Endocrinology, 24, 313-315.

1148. MURAKI, T., TOKUNAGA, Y., MATSUMOTO, S., and MAKINO, T. (1978)
       'Time course of effects of morphine on hypothalamic content
       of LHRH and serum testosterone and LH levels of morphine-
       tolerant and nontolerant male rats.' Archives of Inter-
       national Pharmacodynamics and Therapeutics, 233, 290-295.

1149. MURPHY, M.R. (1981) 'Methadone reduces sexual performances
       and sexual motivation in the male Syrian golden hamster.'
       Pharmacology, Biochemistry, and Behavior, 14, 561-567.

1150. MYERS, B., and BAUM, M. (1979) 'Facilitation by opiate antagon-
       ists of sexual performance in the male rat.' Pharmacology,
       Biochemistry, and Behavior, 10, 615-618.

1151. MYERS, H.B.   (1931)   'Effect of chronic morphine poisoning.'
       Journal of Pharmacology and Experimental Therapeutics,
       41, 317-323.

1152. NEUMAN, L.L.   (1973)   'Drug abuse in pregnancy: Its effects on
       the fetus and newborn infant.'   In: E. Harms, ed. Drugs
       and Youth: The Challenge of Today. Elmsford, New York:
       Pergamon Press.

1153. NORTHROP, G., DITZLER, J., RYAN, W.G., and WILBANKS, G.D.   (1972)
       'Estriol excretion profiles in narcotic-addicted pregnant
       women.'   American Journal of Obstetrics and Gynecology, 112,
       704-712.

1154. ORBAN, P.T.D., and ORBAN, P.T.   (1974)   'A follow-up study of
       female narcotic addicts: Variables related to outcome.'
       British Journal of Psychiatry, 125, 28-33.

1155. OSTROWSKI, N.L., STAPLETON, J.M., NOBLE, R.G., and REID, L.D.
       (1979)   'Morphine and naloxone's effects on sexual behavior
       of the female golden hamster.'   Pharmacology, Biochemistry,
       and Behavior, 11, 673-681.

1156. PACKMAN, P.M., and ROTHCHILD, J.A.   (1976)   'Morphine inhibition
       of ovulation: Reversal by naloxone.'   Endocrinology, 99,
       7-10.

1157. PANG, C.N., ZIMMERMANN, E., and SAWYER, C.   (1974)   'Effects of
       morphine on the surge of luteinizing hormone in the rat.'
       Anatomical Record, 178, 434.

1158. PANTLEO, P.M., and KELLING, G.W.   (1972)   'Quantifiable aspects
       of human figure drawings by male narcotics addicts: Repli-
       cations and extensions.'   Perceptual Motor Skills, 34,
       791-798.

1159. PAROLI, E., and MELCHIORRI, P.   (1961)   'Inhibitory effect of
       morphine on metabolism of adrenal and testicular steroids.'
       Biochemical Pharmacology, 6, 18-20.

1160. PARR, D.   (1976)   'Sexual aspects of drug abuse in narcotic ad-
       dicts.'   British Journal of Addiction, 71, 261-268.

1161. PESCOR, M.J.   (1943)   'A statistical analysis of the clinical
       records of hospitalized drug addicts.'   Public Health
       Reports, Supplement No. 143, 1-30.

1162. PESCOR, M.J.   (1952)   'The problem of narcotic drug addiction.'
       Journal of Criminal Law, Criminology, and Police Science,
       43, 471-481.

1163. PINSKY, C., KOVEN, S.J., and LABELLA, F.S.   (1975)   'Evidence for
       role of endogenous sex steroids in morphine antinociception.'
       Life Sciences, 16, 1785-1786.

1164. PUROHIT, V., SINGH, H.H., and AHLUWALIA, B.S. (1978) 'Failure of methadone-treated human testes to respond to the stimulatory effect of human chorionic gonadotrophin on testosterone biosynthesis in vitro.' Journal of Endocrinology, 78, 299-300.

1165. RADO, S. (1926) 'The psychic effect of intoxicants.' International Journal of Psychoanalysis, 7, 356-413.

1166. RADO, S. (1933) 'The psychoanalysis of pharmacothymia.' Psychiatric Quarterly, 2, 1-23.

1167. REITH, G., CROCKETT, D., and CRAIG, K. (1975) 'Personality characteristics in heroin addicts and nonaddicted prisoners using the Edwards Personality Preference Schedule.' International Journal of the Addictions, 10, 97-112.

1168. RENNELS, E. (1961) 'Effect of morphine on pituitary cytology and gonadotrophic levels in the rat.' Texas Reports on Biology and Medicine, 19, 646-657.

1169. ROSENBAUM, M. (1981) Women on Heroin. New Brunswick, New Jersey: Rutgers University Press.

1170. SANTEN, F.J., SOFSKY, J., EILIC, N., and LIPPERT, R. (1975) 'Mechanism of action of narcotics in the production of menstrual dysfunction in women.' Fertility and Sterility, 26, 538-548.

1171. SAVAGE, C. (1980) 'Sex and heroin.' American Journal of Psychiatry, 137, 951-952.

1172. SAVITT, R.A. (1963) 'Psychoanalytic studies on addiction.' Psychoanalytic Quarterly, 32, 43-57.

1173. SAWYER, C.H., CRITCHLOW, B., and BARRACLOUGH, C.A. (1955) 'Mechanism of blockade of pituitary activation in the rat by morphine, atropine, and barbiturates.' Endocrinology, 57, 345-354.

1174. SCHER, J. (1967) 'Patterns and profiles of addiction and drug abuse.' International Journal of the Addictions, 2, 171-190.

1175. SCHUR, E.M. (1962) Narcotic Addiction in Great Britain and America: The Impact of Public Policy. Bloomington, Indiana: Indiana University Press, pp. 129-130.

1176. SEEVERS, M. (1936) 'Opiate addiction in the monkey. II. Dilaudin in comparison with morphine, heroin, and codeine.' Journal of Pharmacology, 56, 157-165.

1177. SENAY, E., DORUS, W., and RENAULT, P. (1977) 'Methadyl acetate and methadone--an open comparison.' Journal of the American Medical Association, 237, 138-142.

1178.   SHERIDAN, P.J.   (1978)   'Effects of morphine and methadone on the nuclear uptake of estradiol by the brain.'   Clinical Toxicology, 13, 383-390.

1179.   SHOEMAKER, J.V.   (1908)   Materia Medica and Therapeutics.

1180.   SINGH, H.H., PUROHIT, V., and AHLUWALIA, B.S.   (1982)   'Methadone blocks dopamine-mediated release of gonadotropins in rat hypothalamus.'   Neuroendocrinology, 34, 347-352.

1181.   SMITH, D.E., MOSER, C., WESSON, D.R., APTER, M., BUXTON, M.E., DAVISON, J.V., ORGEL, M., and BUFFUM, J.   (1982)   'A clinical guide to the diagnosis and treatment of heroin-related sexual dysfunction.'   Journal of Psychoactive Drugs, 14, 91-99.

1182.   SOYKA, L.F., JOFFE, J.M., and SMITH, S.M.   (1980)   'Influence of concurrent testosterone on the effects of methadone on male rats and their progeny.'   Developmental Pharmacology and Therapeutics, 1, 182-188.

1183.   SOYKA, L.F., PETERSON, J.M., and JOFFE, J.M.   (1978)   'Lethal and sublethal effects on the progeny of male rats treated with methadone.'   Toxicology and Applied Pharmacology, 45, 797-807.

1184.   STOFFER, S.S.   (1968)   'A gynecologic study of drug addicts.'   American Journal of Obstetrics and Gynecology, 101, 779-783.

1185.   STOFFER, S.S., SAPIRA, J.D., and MEKETOR, B.F.   (1965)   'Behavior in ex-addict female prisoners participating in a research study.'   Comprehensive Psychiatry, 10, 224-232.

1186.   SUTKER, P.B., and ALLAIN, A.N.   (1974)   'Addict attitudes toward methadone maintenance: A preliminary report.'   International Journal of the Addictions, 9, 337-343.

1187.   SYLVESTER, P.W., CHEN, H.T., and MEITES, J.   (1980)   'Effects of morphine and naloxone on phasic release of luteinized hormone and follicle-stimulating hormone.'   Proceedings of the Society for Experimental Biology and Medicine, 164, 207-211.

1188.   SYLVESTER, P.W., VAN VUST, D.A., AYLSWORTH, C.A., HANSON, E.A., and MEITES, J.   (1982)   'Effects of morphine and naloxone on inhibition by ovarian hormones of pulsatile release of LH in ovariectomized rats.'   Neuroendocrinology, 34, 269-273.

1189.   TEN HOUTEN, S.   (1982)   'Sexual dynamics and strength of human addiction: A three-factor model of an ideology.'   Journal of Psychoactive Drugs, 14, 101-109.

1190.   TERRY, C.E., and PELLENS, M.   (1928)   The Opium Problem.   Montclair, New Jersey: Patterson Smith.

1191.   THOMAS, J.A., and DOMBROSKY, J.T. (1975) 'Effects of methadone
        on the male reproductive system.' Archives of International
        Pharmacodynamic Therapeutics, 215, 215-221.

1192.   THOMAS, J.A., SHAHID-SALLES, K.S., and DONOVAN, M.P. (1977)
        'Effects of narcotics on the reproductive system.' Advances
        in Sex Hormone Research, 3, 169-195.

1193.   TOKUNAGA, Y., MURAKI, T., and HOSOYA, E. (1977) 'Effects of
        repeated morphine administration on copulation and on the
        hypothalamic-pituitary-gonadal axis of male rats.' Japanese
        Journal of Pharmacology, 27, 65-70.

1194.   TOLIS, G., HICKEY, J., and GUYDA, H. (1975) 'Effects of mor-
        phine on serum growth hormone, cortisol, prolactin, and
        thyroid stimulating hormone in man.' Journal of Clinical
        Endocrinology and Metabolism, 41, 797-800.

1195.   TOYODA, M. (1977) 'Effects of morphine-nitrous oxide anesthesia
        and surgery on plasma levels of luteinizing hormone, testos-
        terone, and cortisol.' Japanese Journal of Anesthesiology,
        26, 279-286.

1196.   VON GRAFFENREID, B., DEL POZO, E., ROUBICEK, J., KREBS, E.,
        POLDINGER, W., BURMEISTER, P., and KERP, L. (1978) 'Ef-
        fects of the synthetic enkephalin analogue FK 33-824 on man.'
        Nature, 272, 729-730.

1197.   WALLACH, R.C., JEREZ, E., and BLINICK, G. (1969) 'Pregnancy and
        menstrual function in narcotic addicts treated with meth-
        adone, the methadone maintenance treatment program.' Amer-
        ican Journal of Obstetrics and Gynecology, 105, 1226-1229.

1198.   WEISS, R.D. (1982) 'Effects of opiates on orgasm.' Medical As-
        pects of Human Sexuality, 16, 29.

1199.   WELLISCH, D., GAY, G., and MC ENTEE, R. (1970) 'The easy rider
        syndrome: A pattern of hetero- and homosexual relationships
        in a heroin addict population.' Family Process, 9, 425-430.

1200.   WESTERMEYER, J., and BERGER, L.J. (1977) '"World Traveler" ad-
        dicts in Asia: I. Demographic and clinical description.'
        American Journal of Drug and Alcohol Abuse, 4, 479-493.

1201.   WHALEY, C.C. (1924) 'The mental and nervous side of addiction
        to narcotic drugs.' Journal of the American Medical Assoc-
        iation, 83, 321-324.

1202.   WIELAND, W., and YUNGER, M. (1971) 'Sexual effects and side ef-
        fects of heroin and methadone.' In: United States Depart-
        ment of Health, Education, and Welfare. Proceedings of the
        Third National Conference on Methadone Treatment, Novem-
        ber 14-16, 1970. Washington, D.C.: U.S. Government Print-
        ing Office; Rockville, Maryland: Public Health Service Pub-
        lication No. 2172, pp. 50-53.

1203. WIKLER, A. (1952) 'A psychodynamic study of a patient during self-regulated readdiction to morphine.' Psychiatric Quarterly, 26, 270-293.

1204. WIKLER, A. (1953) Opiate Addiction. Springfield, Illinois: C.C. Thomas.

1205. WIKLER, A. (1967) 'Opioid addiction.' In: A.M. Freedman and H.I. Kaplan, eds. Comprehensive Textbook of Psychiatry. Baltimore, Maryland: Williams and Wilkins Co., pp. 989-1003.

1206. WIKLER, A. (1971) 'Drug dependence.' In: A. Baker, ed. Clinical Neurology. Volume 2. New York: Harper and Row, pp. 1-42.

1207. WIKLER, A. (1975) 'Drug dependence.' In: A. Baker and L.H. Baker, eds. Clinical Neurology. Hagerstown, Maryland: Harper and Row, pp. 1-61.

1208. WIKLER, A., and RASOR, R. (1953) 'Psychiatric aspects of drug addiction.' American Journal of Medicine, 14, 566-570.

1209. WILLIS, L. (1969) 'Drug dependence: Some demographic and psychiatric aspects in UK and US subjects.' British Journal of Addiction, 64, 135.

1210. WINICK, C., ed. (1974) Sociological Aspects of Drug Dependence. Cleveland, Ohio: CRC Press.

1211. WINICK, C., and KINSIE, P. (1971) The Lively Commerce: Prostitution in the United States. Chicago, Illinois: Quadrangle Books.

1212. WITTON, K. (1962) 'Sexual dysfunction secondary to Mellaril.' Diseases of the Nervous System, 23, 175.

1213. YAFFE, G.J., STRELINGER, R.W., and PARWATIKAR, S. (1973) 'Physical symptom complaints of patients on methadone maintenance.' Proceedings of the National Conference on Methadone Treatment, 1, 507-514.

1214. YORKE, C. (1970) 'A critical review of some psychoanalytic literature on drug addiction.' British Journal of Medical Psychology, 43, 141.

1215. ZIMMERMANN, E., and PANG, C.N. (1976) 'Acute effects of opiate administration on pituitary gonadotropin and prolactin release.' In: D.H. Ford and D.H. Clouet, eds. Tissue Responses to Addictive Drugs. Holliswood, New York: Spectrum Publications, pp. 517-526.

Nitrites

1216. DAHLBERG, C.C. (1976) 'Brief guide to office counseling: When patients ask about amyl nitrite as a sexual stimulant.' Medical Aspects of Human Sexuality, 10, 137.

1217. EVERETT, G.M. (1972) 'Effects of amyl nitrite ("poppers") on sexual experience.' Medical Aspects of Human Sexuality, 6, 146-150.

1218. EVERETT, G.M. (1975) 'Amyl nitrite ("poppers") as an aphrodesiac.' In: M. Sandler and G. Gessa, eds. Sexual Behavior: Pharmacology and Biochemistry. New York: Raven Press, pp. 97-98.

1219. KRAMER, N.D. (1977) 'Availability of volatile nitrites.' Journal of the American Medical Association, 237, 1693.

1220. LABATAILLE, L.M. (1975) 'Amyl nitrite employed in homosexual relations.' Medical Aspects of Human Sexuality, 9, 122.

1221. LOURIA, D.B. (1970) 'Sexual use of amyl nitrite.' Medical Aspects of Human Sexuality, 4, 89 (letter).

1222. LOWRY, T.P. (1979) 'Amyl nitrite: An old high comes back to visit.' Behavioral Medicine, 6, 19-21.

1223. LOWRY, T.P. (1979) 'The volatile nitrites as sexual drugs: A user survey.' Journal of Sexual Education, 1, 8-10.

1224. LOWRY, T.P. (1982) 'Psychosexual aspects of the volatile nitrites.' Journal of Psychoactive Drugs, 14, 77-79.

1225. PERLMAN, J.T., and ADAMS, G.I. (1970) 'Amyl nitrite inhalation fad.' Journal of the American Medical Association, 212, 160 (letter).

1226. SIGELL, L.T., KAPP, F.T., FUSARO, G.A., NELSON, E.D., and
          FALCK, R.S. (1978) 'Popping and snorting volatile
          nitrites: A current fad for getting high.' American
          Journal of Psychiatry, 135, 1216-1218.

1227. WELTI, D.R., and BRODSKY, J. (1980) 'Treatment of intra-
          operative penile tunescence.' Journal of Urology,
          124, 925-926.

1228. LINDER, R.L., LERNER, S.E., and BURNS, R.S. (1981) PCP: The Devil's Dust. Belmont, California: Wadsworth.

1229. SMITH, D.E., SMITH, N., BUXTON, M.E., and MOSER, C. (1980) 'PCP and sexual dysfunction.' Journal of Psychedèlic Drugs, 12, 269-273.

1230. SMITH, D.E., WESSON, D.R., BUXTON, M.E., SEYMOUR, R., and KRAMER, H.M. (1978) 'The diagnosis and treatment of the PCP abuse syndrome.' In: P.C. Petersen and R.C. Stillman, eds. Phencyclidine (PCP) Abuse: An Appraisal. Rockville, Maryland: NIDA Research Monograph.

Tobacco

1231. AFANASSIEV, K.M. (1931) 'Effects of nicotine on the sexual function of man.' Vrachebnaia Gazeta, 35, 1617-1619.

1232. AGAR, W.T. (1940) 'The action of adrenaline upon the uterus of the guinea pig and its modification by eserine.' Journal of Physiology, 98, 492-502.

1233. ALAVERDIAN, A.G., KALANTAROVA, L.G., ARAKELIAN, R.N., and KAZARIAN, L.G. (1976) 'Morphological changes in the uterus and placenta of pregnant rats under the influence of tobacco smoke.' [In Russian.] Zhurnal Eksperimental'noi i Klinicheskoi Meditsiny, 16, 48-52.

1234. ALAVERDIAN, A.G., KALANTAROVA, L.G., ESHCHUTKIN, G.D., KIRAKOSIAN, S.A., and VANETSIAN, A. (1976) 'Morphological changes in the ovaries, adrenals, and pituitary of pregnant rats exposed to tobacco smoke chronically.' [In Russian.] Zhurnal Eksperimental'noi i Klinicheskoi Meditsiny, 16, 48-52.

1235. AMELAR, R.D., DUBIN, L., and SCHOENFELD, C. (1980) 'Sperm motility.' Fertility and Sterility, 34, 197-215.

1236. ANONYMOUS. (1981) 'Smoking and sperm.' Science News, 119, 247.

1237. BAILEY, A., ROBINSON, D., and VESSEY, M. (1977) 'Smoking and age of natural menopause.' Lancet, 2, 722.

1238. BALLANTYNE, J.W. (1902) Manual of Antenatal Pathology and Hygiene: The Fetus. Edinburgh: William Green and Sons.

1239. BEHREND, A., and THIENES, C.H. (1931) 'Failure of nicotine to alter estrus cycle in white rat.' Proceedings of the Society for Experimental Biology and Medicine, 28, 740-741.

1240. BEHREND, A., and THIENES, C.H. (1932) 'Chronic nicotinism in young rats and rabbits: Effect on growth and estrus.' Journal of Pharmacology and Experimental Therapeutics, 46, 113-124.

1241. BEHREND, A., and THIENES, C.H. (1933) 'The development of
      tolerance to nicotine by rats.' Journal of Pharmacology
      and Experimental Therapeutics, 48, 317-325.

1242. BENIGNI, P.F. (1911) 'Sulle alterazioni anatomiche indotte
      dall'intossicazione cronica sperimentale da tabacco.'
      ['Anatomical changes induced by chronic experimental in-
      toxication with tobacco.'] Revista di Patologia Nervosa,
      16, 80-100.

1243. BENZ, J. (1980) 'Female infertility.' Praxis, 69, 1769-1773.

1244. BERRY, E.M. (1981) 'Sperm abnormalities and cigarette smoking.'
      Lancet, 1, 1159.

1245. BETTS, C.A. (1965) 'Smokers seek masculinity.' Science News
      Letter, 87, 373.

1246. BISSET, G.W., and WALKER, J.M. (1957) 'The effects of nicotine,
      hexamethonium, and ethanol on the secretion of the anti-
      diuretic and oxytocic hormones of the rat.' British Journal
      of Pharmacology, 12, 461-467.

1247. BLAKE, C.A. (1974) 'Parallelism and divergence in LH and FSH
      release in nicotince-treated rats.' Proceedings of the
      Society for Experimental Biology and Medicine, 145, 706-
      710.

1248. BLAKE, C.A. (1978) 'Paradoxical effects of drugs acting on the
      central nervous system on the perovulatory release of
      pituitary luteinizing hormone in proestrous rats.'
      Journal of Endocrinology, 79, 319-326.

1249. BLAKE, C.A., NORMAN, R.L., SCARAMUZZI, R.J., and SAWYER, C.H.
      (1973) 'Inhibition of the proestrous surge of prolactin
      in the rat by nicotine.' Endocrinology, 91, 1334-1338.

1250. BLAKE, C.A., and SAWYER, C.H. (1972) 'Nicotine blocks the
      suckling-induced rise in circulating prolactin in lactating
      rats.' Science, 177, 619-621.

1251. BLAKE, C.A., SCARAMUZZI, R.J., NORMAN, R.L., KANEMATSU, S.,
      and SAWYER, C.H. (1972) 'Effect of nicotine on the pro-
      estrus ovulatory surge of LH in the rat.' Endocrinology,
      91, 1253-1258.

1252. BLAKE, C.A., SCARAMUZZI, R.J., NORMAN, R.L., KANEMATSU, S.,
      and SAWYER, C.H. (1972) 'Nicotine delays the ovulatory
      surge of luteinizing hormone in the rat.' Proceedings of
      the Society for Experimental Biology, 141, 1014-1016.

1253. BLOCH, I. (1928) The Sexual Life of Our Time in Its Relation to
      Modern Civilization. New York: Allied Book Company.

1254. BOYCE, A., SCHWARTZ, D., and DAVID, G.   (1976) 'Smoking and
       genitourinary infection.' British Medical Journal, 2, 1013.

1255. BRANCH, H.E., and MOSS, W.G.   (1938) 'Effects of nicotine on
       rats (albino).' Transactions of the Kansas Academy of
       Sciences, 41, 317-329.

1256. BRIGGS, M.H.   (1973) 'Cigarette smoking and infertility in men.'
       Medical Journal of Australia, 7, 616-617.

1257. BUEL, F., BUEL, W., FIELDING, F., LITTLE, D., LITTLE, M., and
       THIENES, C.H.   (1937) 'Estrus and reproduction in the
       white rat as influenced by chronic nicotinism.' Journal
       of Pharmacology and Experimental Therapeutics, 60, 100.

1258. CAMPAGNOLI, C., PRELATO, L., and ROSSETTI, M.G.   (1980) 'Estro-
       gen therapy for the climacteric and thromboembolic risk.'
       Minerva Ginecologia, 32, 429-435.

1259. CAMPBELL, A.M.   (1935) 'Excessive cigarette smoking in women and
       its effect upon their reproductive efficiency.' Journal of
       the Michigan Medical Society, 34, 146-151.

1260. CAMPBELL, A.M.   (1936) 'The effect of excessive cigarette
       smoking on maternal health.' American Journal of Obstetrics
       and Gynecology, 31, 502-508.

1261. CAMPBELL, J.M., and HARRISON, K.L.   (1979) 'Smoking and infer-
       tility.' Medical Journal of Australia, 1, 342-343.

1262. CARNEY, R.E.   (1967) 'Sex chromatin, body masculinity, achieve-
       ment motivation, and smoking behavior.' Psychological
       Reports, 20, 859-866.

1263. CARVER, J.R.   (1981) 'Smoking and sexual functioning.' Medical
       Aspects of Human Sexuality, 15, 13.

1264. CENDRON, H., and VALLERY-MASSON, J.   (1971) 'Tobacco and male
       sexual behavior.' Vie Médicale, 25, 3027-3029.

1265. CHAMBERLAIN, G.   (1981) 'Aetiology of gynaecological cancer.'
       Journal of the Royal Society of Medicine, 74, 246-261.

1266. COLEMAN, S., PIOTROW, P.T., and RINEHART, W.   (1979) Tobacco:
       Hazards to Health and Human Reproduction. Population Re-
       ports, Series L. Baltimore, Maryland: Johns Hopkins Uni-
       versity Population Information Program.

1267. COUDRAY, P.   (1971) 'Tobacco and female sexual behavior.' Vie
       Médicale, 25, 3031-3052.

1268. DANIEL, C., NITZESCU, I.I., SOIMARU, A., and GEORESCU, I.D.   (1935)
      'Recherches expérimentales sur la motilité de la trompe uter-
      ine de la femme.' ['Experimental studies on the motility of
      the female uterus.'] Comptes Rendus des Seances de la
      Société de Biologie, 120, 54-56.

1269. DANIELL, H.W.   (1976) 'Osteoporosis of the slender smoker.'
      Archives of Internal Medicine, 136, 298-304.

1270. DANIELL, H.W.   (1978) 'Smoking, obesity, and the menopause.'
      Lancet, 2, 373.

1271. DATEY, K.K., and DALVI, C.P.   (1972) 'Tobacco and health.' In-
      dian Journal of Chest Diseases, 14, 158-167.

1272. DONTENWILL, W., CHEVALIER, H.-J., HARKE, H.-P., LAFRENZ, U.,
      RECKZEH, G., and SCHNEIDER, B.   (1973) 'Experimental in-
      vestigations of the effect of cigarette smoke exposure on
      testicular function of Syrian golden hamsters.' Toxicology,
      1, 309-320.

1273. DOTSON, L.E., ROBERTSON, L.S., and TUCHFELD, B.   (1975) 'Plasma
      alcohol, smoking, hormone concentrations, and self-reported
      aggression: A study in a social-drinking situation.' Jour-
      nal of Studies on Alcohol, 36, 578-586.

1274. DRAC, P., and KOPECNY, J.   (1970) 'Sterility in female smokers
      and nonsmokers.' Zentralblatt für Gynäkologie, 92, 865-866.

1275. DRIFE, J.O.   (1982) 'Drugs and sperm.' British Medical Jour-
      nal, 284, 844.

1276. DRYSDALE, C.R.   (1975) 'Tobacco, and its effects on the health
      of males.' British Medical Journal, 2, 271.

1277. EDMUNDS, C.W.   (1920) 'The point of attack of certain drugs
      acting on the retractor penis muscle of the dog.' Journal
      of Pharmacology and Experimental Therapeutics, 15, 201-216.

1278. ENEROTH, P., FUXE, K., GUSTAFSSON, J.-A., HÖKFELT, T., LÖF-
      STRÖM, A., SKETT, P., and AGNATI, L.   (1977) 'The effect of
      nicotine on central catecholamine neurons and gonadotropin
      secretion. II. Inhibitory influence of nicotine on LH, FSH,
      and prolactin secretion in the ovariectomized female rat and
      its relation to regional changes in dopamine and noradren-
      aline levels and turnover.' Medical Biology, 55, 158-166.

1279. ENEROTH, P., FUXE, K., GUSTAFSSON, J.-A., HÖKFELT, T., LÖF-
      STRÖM, A., SKETT, P., and AGNATI, L.   (1977) 'The effect of
      nicotine on central catecholamine neurons and gonadotropin
      secretion. III. Studies on prepubertal female rats treated
      with pregnant mare serum gonadotropin.' Medical Biology, 55,
      167-176.

1280. ERBACHER, K,, GRUMBRECHT, P., and LÖSER, A. (1940) 'Nikotin und
       innere Sekretion.' ['Nicotine and inner secretion.'] Archiv
       für Experimentelle Pathologie und Pharmakologie, 195, 121-
       142.

1281. ESSENBERG, J.M., FAGAN, L., and MALERSTEIN, A.J. (1951) 'Chronic
       poisoning of the ovaries and testes of albino rats and mice
       by nicotine and cigarette smoke.' Western Journal of Sur-
       gery, Obstetrics, and Gynecology, 59, 27-32.

1282. EVANS, H.J., FLETCHER, J., TORRANCE, M., and HARGREAVE, T.B.
       (1981) 'Sperm abnormalities and cigarette smoking.' Lan-
       cet, 1, 627-629.

1283. FARRELL, J.I., and LYMAN, Y. (1937) 'A study of the secretory
       nerves of, and the action of certain drugs on, the prostate
       gland.' American Journal of Physiology, 118, 64-70.

1284. FERRY, J.D., MC LEAN, B.K., and NIKITOVITCH-WINER, M.B. (1974)
       'Tobacco-smoke inhalation delays suckling-induced prolactin
       release in the rat.' Proceedings of the Society for Ex-
       perimental Biology and Medicine, 147, 110-113.

1285. FORSBERG, L., GUSTAVII, B., HOJERBACK, T., and OLSSON, A.M.
       (1979) 'Impotence, smoking, and beta-blocking drugs.' Fer-
       tility and Sterility, 31, 589-591.

1286. FRANZ, K. (1904) 'Studien zur Phyiologie des Uterus.' ['Studies
       on the physiology of the uterus.'] Zeitschrift für Geburts-
       hilfe und Gynäkologie, 53, 361-419.

1287. FRETS, G.P. (1930) 'Keimgifte.' ['Germ poisoning.'] Archivio
       e Rassegna Italiana di Ottalmologia, 24, 91-92.

1288. FUXE, K., AGNATI, L., ENEROTH, P., GUSTAFSSON, J.-A., HÖKFELT, T.,
       LÖFSTRÖM, A., SKETT, B., and SKETT, P. (1977) 'The effect
       of nicotine on central catecholamine neurons and gonado-
       tropin secretion. I. Studies in the male rat.' Medical
       Biology, 55, 148-157.

1289. FUXE, K., EVERITT, B.J., and HÖKFELT, T. (1979) 'Enhancement
       of sexual behavior in the female rat by nicotine. Pharma-
       cology, Biochemistry, and Behavior, 7, 147-151.

1290. GODFREY, B. (1981) 'Sperm morphology in smokers.' Lancet, 1,
       948.

1291. GORDON, B. (1981) 'Sperm morphology in smokers.' Lancet, 1,
       948.

1292. GRUMBRECHT, P., and LÖSER, A. (1940) 'Nikotin und innere Se-
      kretion. II. Arbeitsschaden der Frau in Tabakfabriken?'
      ['Nicotine and internal secretion. II. Work-related damage
      among women employed in the tobacco industry?'] Archiv für
      Experimentelle Pathologie und Pharmakologie, 195, 143-151.

1293. GRUMBRECHT, P., and LÖSER, A. (1941) 'Nikotin und innere Se-
      kretion: Erbpathologische Untersuchungen über Keimschadig-
      ungen durch Nikotin.' ['Nicotine and internal secretion:
      Pathological study of germ poisoning by nicotine.'] Klin-
      ische Wochenschrift, 2, 853-858.

1294. HAGSTROM, B.E., and ALLEN, R.D. (1956) 'The mechanism of
      nicotine-induced polyspermy.' Experimental Cell Research,
      10, 14-23.

1295. HASAMA, B. (1933) 'Recherches pharmacologiques sur le courant
      electrique au conduit spermatique isole.' ['Pharmacological
      studies on electrical current in the motility of isolated
      sperm.'] Japanese Journal of Medical Science and Pharma-
      cology, 7, 81-82.

1296. HEMSWORTH, B.N. (1978) 'Embryopathies due to nicotine referable
      to impairment of spermatogenesis in the mouse.' IRCS Med-
      ical Sciences Library Compendium, 6, 461.

1297. HEMSWORTH, B.N., and WARDHAUGH, A.A. (1976) 'Antifertility
      action of nicotine in the male mouse.' IRCS Medical
      Sciences Library Compendium, 4, 519.

1298. HENDERSON, V.E., and ROEPKE, M.H. (1933) 'On the mechanism of
      erection.' American Journal of Physiology, 106, 441-448.

1299. HEYER. G.R. (1939) 'Smoking and sexual impotence.' Münchener
      Medizinische Wochenschrift, 86, 1132.

1300. HOFSTATTER, R. (1923) 'Experimentelle Studien über die Ein-
      wirkung des Nikotins auf die Keimdrusen und auf die Fort-
      pflanzung.' ['Experimental studies on the effects of
      nicotine on the gonads and on reproduction.'] Virchow's
      Archives für Pathologie und Anatomie, 244, 183-213.

1301. HOLSTE, A. (1924) 'Untersuchungen am überlebenden Uterus.'
      ['Examination of the enlarged uterus.'] Archives für
      Experimentelle Pathologie und Pharmakologie, 101, 36-53.

1302. HOTOVY, R. (1948) 'Versuche zur Frage des Einflusses der
      chronischen Nikotinschädigung auf Fruchtbarkeit und Nach-
      kommenschaft.' ['Experiments to determine the effect of
      chronic exposure to nicotine upon fertility and subsequent
      progeny.'] Naunyn-Schmiedeberg's Archives of Pathology,
      205, 54-56.

1303.   HUDSON, D.B., and TIMIRAS, P.S.   (1972)   'Nicotine injection
            during gestation: Impairment of reproduction, fetal via-
            bility, and development.'   Biology of Reproduction, 7, 247-
            253.

1304.   JICK, H., PORTER, J., and MORRISON, A.S.   (1977)   'Relation
            between smoking and age of natural menopause.'   Lancet, 1,
            1354-1355.

1305.   JOHNS, W.S.   (1944)   'Tobacco, drug and delight.'   Historical
            Bulletin, 9, 23-31.

1306.   JOSEPH, OF CUPERTINO.   (1718)   At the Congregation of Sacred Rites
            on the Beatification and Canonization of the Venerable Ser-
            vant of God, Joseph a Cupertino, Professed Priest of the
            Lesser Conventual Order of St. Francis (sponsored by) the
            Most Eminent and Reverend Lord Cardinal Casini of Nardo.
            Responses of Fact and of Law to the Objections of the Rever-
            end Father, the Advancer of Truth, Concerning the Doubt
            Whether He Possesses the Theological Virtues: Faith, Hope,
            and Charity, and the Cardinal Virtues: Prudence, Justice,
            Fortitude, and Temperance, and Instances of His Heroic
            Standing in Each Case.   Rome: Apostolic Camera.

1307.   KANEMATSU, S., and SAWYER, C.H.   (1973)   'Inhibition of the
            progesterone-advanced LH surge at proestrus by nicotine.'
            Proceedings of the Society for Experimental Biology and
            Medicine, 143, 1183-1186.

1308.   KAUFMAN, D.W., SLONE, D., ROSENBERG, L., MIETTINEN, O.S., and
            SHAPIRO, S.   (1980)   'Cigarette smoking and age at natural
            menopause.'   American Journal of Public Health, 70, 420-422.

1309.   KEHRER, E.   (1907)   'Physiologische und pharmakologische Unter-
            suchungen an den überlebenden und lebenden inneren Genital-
            ien.'   ['Physiological and pharmacological inquiries of
            longevity and genital function.']   Archiv für Gynäkologie,
            81, 160-210.

1310.   KINGE, E.   (1970)   'The effect of some substances on the isolated
            bull retractor penis muscle.'   Acta Physiologica Scandin-
            avica, 78, 280-288.

1311.   LALL, K.B., SINGHI, S., GURNANI, M., SINGHI, P., and GARG, O.P.
            (1980)   'Somatotype, physical growth, and sexual maturation
            in young male smokers.'   Journal of Epidemiology and
            Community Health, 34, 295-298.

1312.   LARSON, P.S., HAAG, M.B., and SYLVETTE, H.   (1961)   Tobacco:
            Experimental and Clinical Studies.   Baltimore, Maryland:
            Williams and Wilkins Co.,

1313.   LARSON, P.S., and SILVETTE, H., eds.   (1968)   Tobacco: Exper-
            imental and Clinical Studies.   A Comprehensive Account of
            World Literature.   Supplement.   Baltimore, Maryland:
            Williams and Wilkins Co.

1314.   LARSON, P.S., and SILVETTE, H., eds. (1971) Tobacco: Exper-
        imental and Clinical Studies. A Comprehensive Account of
        World Literature. Supplement II. Baltimore, Maryland:
        Williams and Wilkins.

1315.   LARSON, P.S., and SILVETTE, H., eds. (1975) Tobacco: Exper-
        imental and Clinical Studies. A Comprehensive Account of
        World Literature. Supplement III. Baltimore, Maryland:
        Williams and Wilkins.

1316.   LEE, Y.C. (1935) 'Experimental studies on the relation between
        nicotine and sexual hormone. Part I. Lethal dose of
        nicotine and sexual difference.' Journal of the Severance
        Union Medical College, 2, 80-86.

1317.   LEE, Y.C. (1935) 'Experimental studies on the relation between
        nicotine and sexual hormone. Part II: Effect of castration
        and sexual hormone on nicotine toxicity.' Journal of the
        Severance Union Medical College, 2, 87-107.

1318.   LEE, Y.C. (1935) 'Experimental studies on the relation between
        nicotine and sexual hormone. Part III. The effects of
        nicotine on the morphological and histological changes of
        female sexual organs after injections of female sexual
        hormone.' Journal of the Severance Union Medical College,
        2, 108-155.

1319.   LEE, Y.C. (1935) 'Experimental studies on the relation between
        nicotine and sexual hormone. Part IV. The antidotal action
        of luteohormone on nicotine toxicity during anaphylaxis.'
        Journal of the Severance Union Medical College, 2, 156-159.

1320.   LEE, Y.C. (1935) 'The effect of nicotine on sex and sexual
        hormone.' [In Japanese.] Chosen Igaku-Kwai Zasshi, 25,
        716-724.

1321.   LICKINT, F. (1934) 'Der Tabak als Keimgift.' ['Tobacco as
        germ poison.'] Gesundheit und Erziehung, 47, 35-38.

1322.   LINDQUIST, O., and BENGTSSON, C. (1979) 'Menopausal age in
        relation to smoking.' Acta Medica Scandinavica, 205,
        73-77.

1323.   LINDQUIST, O., and BENGTSSON, C. (1979) 'The effect of smoking
        on menopausal age.' Maturitas, 1, 171-173.

1324.   LUCAS, R.C. (1882) 'Underdeveloped testes associated with early
        tobacco-chewing.' British Medical Journal, 2, 889.

1325.   MALCOLM, S., and SHEPHARD, R.J. (1978) 'Personality and sexual
        behavior of the adolescent smoker.' American Journal of
        Drug and Alcohol Abuse, 5, 87-96.

1326. MARTIN-BOYCE, A., DAVID, G., and SCHWARTZ, D. (1977) 'Alcool, tabac et infections genito-urinaires masculines.' ['Alcohol, tobacco, and genitourinary infections in the male.'] Revue d'Epidemiologie et de Santé Publique, 25, 209-216.

1327. MARTINS, T., and VALLE, J.R. (1938) 'Contractilité, survie et pharmacologie in vitro de l'epididyme humain.' ['Contractility, survival, and pharmacology in vitro of the human epididymus.'] Comptes Rendus des Seances de la Société de Biologie, 129, 1152-1155.

1328. MARTINS, T., and VALLE, J.R. (1938) 'Pharmacologie comparée des canaux deferents et des vesicules seminales, in vitro, de rats normaux et de rats castrés.' ['Comparative pharmacology of the different ducts and seminal vesicles of normal and castrated rats, in vitro.'] Comptes Rendus des Seances de la Société de Biologie, 127, 1381-1384.

1329. MARTINS, T., VALLE, J.R., and PORTO, A. (1938) 'Contractilité et reactions pharmacologiques des canaux deferents et des vesicules seminales in vitro, de rats castrés et traites par les hormones sexuelles.' ['Contractility and pharmacological responses of the different ducts and seminal vesicles of castrated rats stimulated by sexual hormones in vitro.'] Comptes Rendus des Seances de la Société de Biologie, 127, 1385-1388.

1330. MARTINS, T., VALLE, J.R., and PORTO, A. (1940) 'Pharmacology in vitro of the human vasa deferentia and epididymus: The question of the endocrine control of the motility of the male accessory genitals.' Journal of Urology, 44, 682-698.

1331. MC KENNEY, F.D., ESSEX, H.E., and MANN, F.C. (1932) 'The action of certain drugs on the oviduct of the domestic fowl.'] Journal of Pharmacology and Experimental Therapeutics, 45, 113-119.

1332. MC LEAN, B.K., RUBEL, A., and NIKITOVITCH-WINER, M.B. (1977) 'The differential effects of exposure to tobacco smoke on the secretion of luteinizing hormone and prolactin in the proestrous rat.' Endocrinology, 100, 1561-1570.

1333. MELLAN, J. (1963) 'Smoking and male sexual defects.' Prakticke Zubni Lekarstvi, 43, 862-863.

1334. MELLAN, J. (1967) 'Smoking and male fertility.' Prakticke Zubni Lekarstvi, 47, 890-892.

1335. MGALOBELI, M. (1931) 'Einfluss der Arbeit in der Tabakindustrie auf die Geschlechtssphäre der Arbeiterin.' ['Influence of work in tobacco industry on reproduction of female workers.'] Monatsschrift der Geburtshilfe und Gynäkologie, 88, 237-247.

1336. NAKAZAWA, R.   (1931)   'Der Einfluss der chronischen Nikotinver-
       giftung auf die Geschlechtsfunktion der weiglichen Ratten.'
       ['Influence of chronic nicotine poisoning on sexual function
       of male rats.']   Japanese Journal of Medical Science, 5, 109-
       111.

1337. NAKAZAWA, R.   (1933)   'Der Einfluss der chronischen Nikotinver-
       giftung auf die Funktion der Geschlechtsorgane der weib-
       lichen Ratten.'   ['Influence of chronic nicotine poisoning
       on the function of the sex organs in the female rat.']
       Japanese Journal of Medical Science, 1, 1-37.

1338. NERI, A., and MARCUS, S.L.   (1972)   'Effect of nicotine on the
       motility of the oviducts in the rhesus monkey: A preliminary
       report.'   Journal of Reproduction and Fertility, 31, 91-97.

1339. OCHSNER, A.   (1971)   'Influence of smoking on sexuality and
       pregnancy.'   Medical Aspects of Human Sexuality, 5, 81-92.

1340. OCHSNER, A.   (1971)   'The health menace of tobacco.'   American
       Scientist, 59, 246-252.

1341. OGATA, S.   (1919)   'Preliminary report of studies on the influence
       of alcohol and nicotine upon the ovary.'   Journal of Medical
       Research, 40, 123-127.

1342. OLSSON, A.M.   (1982)   'Cigarette-induced impotence.'   Medical
       Aspects of Human Sexuality, 16, 13.

1343. PETIT, G.   (1902)   'Les alterations des organes de la génération
       sous l'influence du tabac.'   ['Changes in reproductive organs
       under the influence of tobacco.']   Archives Générales de
       Médicine, 1, 392-394.

1344. PETTERSSON, F.   (1971)   'Medicinska skadeverkningar av rokning:
       Rokning och gynekologisk-obstetriska tillstand.'   ['Adverse
       clinical effects of smoking: Smoking and gynecological-
       obstetrical condition.']   Social-Medicinsk Tidskrift, 2,
       78-82.

1345. PETTERSSON, F.   (1972)   'Rokning och gynekologisk-obstetriske
       tillstand.'   ['Smoking and gynelogical-obstetrical con-
       dition.']   Sykepleien, 59, 68-70.

1346. PETTERSON, F., FRIES, H., and NILLIUS, S.   (1973)   'Epidemiology
       of secondary amenorrhea. I. Incidence and prevalence rates.'
       American Journal of Obstetrics and Gynecology, 117, 80-86.

1347. RABOCH, J., and MELLAN, J.   (1975)   'Smoking and fertility.'
       British Journal of Sexual Medicine, 2, 35, 37.

1348.   SCHINZ, H.R., and SLOTOPOLSKY, B.   (1921)   'Bemerkungen über
        Entwicklung und Pathologie des Hodens.' ['Observations on
        the development and pathology of the testicle.'] Virchows
        Archives Abteilung. Part A: Pathologische Anatomie, 253,
        413-420.

1349.   SCHIRREN, C.   (1970)   'Die kinderlose Ehe: Möglichkeiten und
        Grenzen der Behandlung aus andrologischer Sicht.' ['The
        childless marriage: Possibilities and limitations of the
        treatment from the andrological viewpoint.'] Fortschritte
        der Medizin, 88, 1047-1051.

1350.   SCHIRREN, C.   (1972)   'Die Wirkung des Nikotins auf die Zeugungs-
        fähigkeit des Mannes.' ['The effect of nicotine on the
        procreative ability of the male.'] Rehabilitation, Prä-
        ventivmedizin, Physikalische Medizin, Sozialmedizin, 25,
        23-24.

1351.   SCHIRREN, C.   (1973)   'Importance of follow-up studies in
        andrology.' In: T. Hasegawa, M. Hayashi, F.J.G. Ebling, and
        I.W. Henderson, eds. Fertility and Sterility. New York:
        American Elsevier Publishing Company, pp. 210-213.

1352.   SCHIRREN, C.   (1973)   'Umweltschaden und Fertilität des Mannes:
        Schädigende exogene Einflüsse.' ['Environmental influences
        and fertility of the male: Negative exogenous influences.']
        Andrologie, 5, 91-104.

1353.   SCHIRREN, C.   (1974)   'Andrologische Aspekte der Sterilität.'
        ['Andrological aspects of sterility.'] Gynäkologische
        Rundschau, 14 (Supplement 1), 81-90.

1354.   SCHIRREN, C., and GEY, G.   (1969)   'Der Einfluss des Rauchens auf
        die Fortpflanzungsfähigkeit bei Mann und Frau.' ['The in-
        fluence of smoking on the reproductive ability of men and
        women.'] Zeitschrift für Haut und Geschlechtskrankheiten,
        44, 175-182.

1355.   SELTZER, C.C.   (1959)   'Masculinity and smoking.' Science, 130,
        1706-1707.

1356.   SODANO, A.   (1934)   'Ricerche sperimentali sull' influenza della
        nicotina sulla funzione genitale della donna.' ['Experimen-
        tal study of the influence of nicotine on female sexual func-
        tion.'] Archivio di Ostetricia e Ginecologia, 21, 559-569.

1357.   SOULAIRAC, M.L., and SOULAIRAC, A.   (1972)   'Effect of nicotine
        on the sexual behavior of the male rat.' Comptes Rendus
        des Sciences de la Societe de Biologie, 166, 798-802.

1358.   STADTLANDER, K.H.   (1936)   'Über die Wirkung des Nikotins auf
        Reimdrusen und Nebennieren.' ['Concerning the effects of
        nicotine on glands and adrenals.'] Zeitschrift für die
        Gesamte Experimentelle Medizin, 99, 670-680.

1359. STEKHUN, F.I. (1979) 'Alkogol i tabkourniye kak vozmozhnye prichiny besplodiya muzhchin.' ['Alcohol and tobacco smoking as possible causes of sterility in males.'] Vestnik Dermatologii i Venerologii, 7, 61-65.

1360. STERLING, T.D., and KOBAYASKI, D. (1975) 'A critical review of reports on the effects of smoking on sex and fertility.' Journal of Sex Research, 11, 201-217.

1361. SUBAK-SHARPE, G. (1974) 'Is your sex life going up in smoke?' Today's Health, 52, 50-53.

1362. THIENES, C.H. (1931) 'Failure of nicotine to alter the estrus cycle in the white rat.' Proceedings of the Society for Experimental Biology and Medicine, 28, 740-741.

1363. THIENES, C.H. (1960) 'Chronic nicotine poisoning.' Annals of the New York Academy of Science, 90, 239-248.

1364. THIENES, C.H., LOMBARD, C.F., FIELDING, F.J., LESSER, A.J., and ELLENHORN, M.J. (1946) 'Alterations in reproductive functions of white rats associated with daily exposure to nicotine.' Journal of Pharmacology and Experimental Therapeutics, 87, 1-10.

1365. THOA, N.B., and MAENGWYN-DAVIES, G.D. (1968) 'The guinea-pig isolated vas deferens: A method for increasing sensitivity to drugs.' Journal of Pharmaceutics and Pharmacology, 20, 873-876.

1366. TOKUHATA, G. (1968) 'Smoking in relation to infertility and fetal loss.' Archives of Environmental Health, 17, 353-359.

1367. TOURNADE, A., CHEVILLOT, M., and BERNOT, E. (1938) 'Sur certains troubles due fonctionnement nerveux engendres par l'inhalation de fumée de tabac: Suppression momentanée de la reflectivité tendineuse et de l'excitabilité des nerfs erecteurs.' ['On certain problems of nervous function engendered by the inhalation of tobacco smoke: Momentary suppression of the tendon reflex and the excitability of the erector nerves.'] Comptes Rendus des Seances de la Société de Biologie, 128, 787-789.

1368. UNBEHAUN, G. (1931) 'Untersuchungen über die Einwirkung des Nikotins auf das Ovarius des weissen Maus.' ['Examination of the effects of nicotine on the ovary of the white mouse.'] Archiv für Gynäkologie, 147, 371-383.

1369. UNITED STATES PUBLIC HEALTH SERVICE. (1964) Smoking and Health. Report of the Advisory Committee to the Surgeon General of the Public Health Service. Department of Health, Education, and Welfare, DHEW Publication No. 1103, Washington, D.C.

1370.   UNITED STATES PUBLIC HEALTH SERVICE.   (1971)   The Health Conse-
        sequences of Smoking. A Report of the Surgeon General.
        Department of Health, Education, and Welfare, DHEW Publi-
        cation No. (HSM) 71-7513, Washington, D.C.

1371.   UNITED STATES PUBLIC HEALTH SERVICE.   (1972)   The Health Conse-
        quences of Smoking. A Report of the Surgeon General.
        Department of Health, Education, and Welfare. DHEW Publi-
        cation No. (HSM) 72-7516, Washington, D.C.

1372.   UNITED STATES PUBLIC HEALTH SERVICE.   (1973)   The Health Conse-
        quences of Smoking. A Report of the Surgeon General.
        Department of Health, Education, and Welfare. DHEW Publi-
        cation No. (HSM) 73-8704, Washington, D.C.

1373.   UNITED STATES PUBLIC HEALTH SERVICE.   (1976)   The Health Conse-
        quences of Smoking. A Report of the Surgeon General.
        Department of Health, Education, and Welfare. DHEW Publi-
        cation No. (CDC) 76-8704, Washington D.C.

1374.   UNITED STATED PUBLIC HEALTH SERVICE.   (1979)   Smoking and Health:
        A Report of the Surgeon General. Department of Health,
        Education, and Welfare. DHEW Publication No. (PHS) 79-50066,
        Washington, D.C.

1375.   UNITED STATES PUBLIC HEALTH SERVICE.   (1980)   The Health Conse-
        quences of Smoking for Women: A Report of the Surgeon
        General. U.S. Department of Health and Human Services.
        Office on Smoking and Health, Rockville, Maryland.

1376.   VAN KEEP, P.A., BRAND, P.C., and LEHERT, P. (1979) 'Factors
        affecting the age at menopause.' Journal of Biosocial
        Science, 6 (Supplement), 37-55.

1377.   VESSEY, M.P., WRIGHT, N.H., MC PHERSON, K., and WIGGINS, P.
        (1978) 'Fertility after stopping different methods of con-
        traception.' British Medical Journal, 1, 265-267.

1378.   VICZIAN, M. (1968) 'Dohanyosokon vegzett ondovizsgalatok
        tapasztalatai.' ['Experiences with the sperm of smokers.']
        Orvosi Hetilap, 109, 1077-1079.

1379.   VICZIAN, M. (1968) 'The effect of cigarette smoke inhalation
        on spermatogenesis in the rat.' Experientia, 24, 511-512.

1380.   VICZIAN, M. (1969) 'Ergebnisse von Spermauntersuchungen bei
        Zigarettenrauchern.' ['Results of spermatozoa studies in
        cigarette smokers.'] Zeitschrift für Haut und Geschlechts-
        krankheiten, 44, 183-187.

1381.   VICZIAN, M., and HEINISCH, P. (1967) 'A dohanyzas hatasa a
        spermatogenesisre.' ['The effects of smoking on spermato-
        genesis.'] Magyar Noorvosok Lapja, 35, 412-418.

1382. VON HOFSTATTER, R. (1923) 'Experimentelle Studie über die Ein-
      wirkung des Nikotins auf die Keimdrusen und auf die Fort-
      pflanzung.' ['Experimental studies on the effects of nico-
      tine on the gonads and on propagation.'] Virchows Archiv
      Abteilung. Part A. Pathologische Anatomie und Physiologie,
      244, 183-213.

1383. VON STAMMLER, M. (1935) 'Die chronische Vergiftung mit Nikotin.'
      ['Chronic poisoning with nicotine.'] Virchows Archiv Ab-
      teilung. Part A. Pathologische Anatomie und Physiologie,
      295, 366-393.

1384. VON STAMMLER, M. (1936) 'Nikotin und Keimdrusen.' ['Nicotine
      and the gonads.'] Münchener Medizinische Wochenschrift, 83,
      658.

1385. WADDELL, J.A. (1917) 'The pharmacology of the seminal vesicles.'
      Journal of Pharmacology and Experimental Therapeutics, 9,
      113-120.

1386. WADDELL, J.A. (1917) 'The pharmacology of the uterus masculinus.'
      Journal of Pharmacology and Experimental Therapeutics, 9,
      171-178.

1387. WADDELL, J.A. (1917) 'The pharmacology of the vagina.' Journal
      of Pharmacology and Experimental Therapeutics, 9, 411-426.

1388. WEATHERSBEE, P.S. (1980) 'Nicotine and its influence on the
      female reproductive system.' Journal of Reproductive
      Medicine, 25, 243-250.

1389. WELLBAND, W.A., MINER, N., and STEINHAUS, A.H. (1957) 'Effect
      of tobacco smoke on the artificially induced vaginal
      cycle in spayed rats.' Federation Proceedings; Federation
      of the American Society for Experimental Biology, 16, 136.

1390. WILLENBRECHER, T. (1979) 'Why the Turk can't get it up.' Mother
      Jones, 4, 37-38.

1391. WINTER, R. (1980) 'Hormones and tobacco smoke--when mixed it's
      all ill wind.' Science Digest, 88, 51-58.

1392. WINTERNITZ, W.W., and QUILLEN, D. (1977) 'Acute hormonal
      response to cigarette smoking.' Journal of Clinical
      Pharmacology, 17, 389-397.

1393. WOOD, C., LARSEN, L., and WILLIAMS, R. (1979) 'Duration of
      menstruation.' Australian and New Zealand Journal of Ob-
      stetrics and Gynecology, 19, 216-229.

1394. WOOD, C., LARSEN, L., and WILLIAMS, R. (1979) 'Social and
      psychological factors in relation to premenstrual tension
      and menstrual pain.' Australian and New Zealand Journal
      of Obstetrics and Gynaecology, 19, 111-115.

1395. YUN, I.S., and LEE, Y.S.   (1935)   'Experimental studies on the
      relation between nicotine and sexual hormone.'   Folia Endo-
      crinology Japan, 11, 9-12.

General Reviews

1396. AMERICAN MEDICAL ASSOCIATION COMMITTEE ON HUMAN SEXUALITY. (1972) Human Sexuality. Chicago, Illinois: American Medical Association.

1397. BEAUMONT, G. (1976) 'Untoward effects of drugs on sexuality.' In: S. Crown, ed. Psychosexual Problems: Psychotherapy, Counseling, and Behavioral Modification. London: Academic Press, pp. 325-335.

1398. BRECHER, E.M. (1972) Licit and Illicit Drugs: The Consumers Union Report on Narcotics, Stimulants, Depressants, Inhalants, Hallucinogens, and Marijuana--Including Caffeine, Nicotine, and Alcohol. Boston, Massachusetts: Little, Brown, and Co.

1399. BUFFUM, J. (1982) 'Pharmacosexology: The effects of drugs on sexual function. A review.' Journal of Psychoactive Drugs, 14, 5-44.

1400. BUFFUM, J., SMITH, D.E., MOSER, C., APTER, M., BUXTON, M., and DAVISON, J. (1981) 'Drugs and sexual function.' In: H.J. Lief, ed. Sexual Problems in Medical Practice. Monroe, Wisconsin: American Medical Association, pp. 211-242.

1401. BUSH, P.J. (1980) Drugs, Alcohol, and Sex. New York: Richard Marek.

1402. CANADIAN GOVERNMENT COMMISSION OF INQUIRY. (1971) The Non-Medical Use of Drugs: Interim Report. Baltimore, Maryland: Penguin Books.

1403. COHEN, S. (1981) The Substance Abuse Problems. New York: Haworth Press.

1404. ELLENWOOD, E., and ROCKWELL, W.J. (1975) 'Effect of drug use on sexual behavior.' Medical Aspects of Human Sexuality, 9, 10-32.

1405.   ELLENWOOD, E., and ROCKWELL, W.J.   (1975)   'Effect of drug use
        on sexual behavior.'   Medical Aspects of Human Sexuality, 9,
        10-32.

1406.   FORD, C.S., and BEACH, F.A.   (1951)   Patterns of Sexual Behav-
        ior.   New York: Ace Books.

1407.   FORT, J.   (1975)   'Sex and drugs: The interaction of two
        disapproved behaviors.'   Postgraduate Medicine, 58, 133-
        136.

1408.   FREEDMAN, A.M.   (1976)   'Drugs and sexual behavior.'   In:
        B.J. Sadock, H.I. Kaplan, and A.M. Freedman, eds.   The
        Sexual Experience.   Baltimore, Maryland: Williams and
        Wilkins, pp. 328-334.

1409.   GAWIN, F.H.   (1978)   'Drugs and Eros: Reflections on aphro-
        disiacs.'   Journal of Psychedelic Drugs, 10, 227-236.

1410.   GOTTLIEB, A.   (1975)   Sex Drugs and Aphrodisiacs: Where to
        Obtain Them, How to Use Them, and Their Effects.   New York
        and San Francisco: High Times/Level.

1411.   HIGH TIMES ENCYCLOPEDIA OF RECREATIONAL DRUGS.   (1978)   New York:
        Stonehill Press.

1412.   HOLLISTER, L.   (1975)   'Drugs and sexual behavior in men.'
        Psychopharmacology Bulletin, 11, 44.

1413.   HOLLISTER, L.   (1975)   'The mystique of social drugs and sex.'
        In: M. Sandler and G.L. Gessa, eds.   Sexual Behavior--
        Pharmacology and Biochemistry.   New York: Raven Press,
        pp. 85-92.

1414.   HOROWITZ, J.D., and GOBLE, A.J.   (1979)'   'Drugs and impaired
        male sexual function.'   Drugs, 18, 206-217.

1415.   JONES, H.B., and JONES, H.C.   (1977)   Sensual Drugs: Depri-
        vation and Rehabilitation of the Mind.   Cambridge: Cam-
        bridge University Press.

1416.   KAPLAN, H.S.   (1979)   Disorders of Sexual Desire.   New York:
        Simon and Schuster.

1417.   KAPLAN, H.S.   (1974)   The New Sex Therapy.   New York: Brun-
        ner/Mazel Publishers.

1418.   KATCHADOURIAN, H.A., and LUNDE, D.T.   (1975)   Fundamentals of
        Human Sexuality.   New York: Holt, Rinehart, and Winston.

1419.   KOLODNY, R.C., MASTERS, W.H., and JOHNSON, V.E.   (1979)   Text-
        book of Sexual Medicine.   Boston, Massachusetts: Little,
        Brown, and Co.

1420.   LEAVITT, F. (1982) Drugs and Behavior. New York: John Wiley
         and Sons.

1421.   MANN, T.   (1968) 'Effects of pharmacological agents on male
         sexual functions.' Journal of Reproduction and Fertility,
         4 (Supplement), 101-114.

1422.   MUNJACK, D.J. (1979) 'Sex and drugs.' Clinical Toxicology,
         15, 75-89.

1423.   NOWLIS, V. (1975) 'Categories of interest in the scientific
         search for relationships (i.e., interactions, associations,
         comparisons) in human sexual behavior and drug use.' In:
         M. Sandler and G.L. Gessa, eds. Sexual Behavior: Pharm-
         acology and Biochemistry. New York: Raven Press, pp. 93-
         96.

1424.   PIEMIME, T. (1976) 'Sex and illicit drugs.' Medical Aspects
         of Human Sexuality, 10, 85-86.

1425.   RENSHAW, D.C. (1978) 'Sex and drugs.' South Africa Medical
         Journal, 54, 322-326.

1426.   SELDEN, G. (1979) Aphrodisia. New York: E.P. Dutton.

1427.   SHOCHET, B.R. (1976) 'Medical aspects of sexual dysfunctions.'
         Drug Therapy, 6, 37-42.

1428.   WATTS, R.J. (1978) 'The physiological interrelationships
         between depression, drugs, and sexuality.' Nursing Forum,
         17, 168-183.

1429.   WHITLOCK, F.A. (1979) Drugs, Drinking, and Recreational Drug
         Use in Australia. New South Wales, Australia: Cassell
         Australia.

1430.   WILSON, R.A. (1973) Sex and Drugs. Chicago, Illinois:
         Playboy Press.

1431.   WITTERS, W.L., and JONES-WITTERS, P. (1975) Drugs and Sex.
         New York and London: Macmillan/Collier-Macmillan.

1432.   WOODS, J. (1975) 'Drug effects in human sexual behavior.'
         In: N.F. Woods, ed. Human Sexuality in Health and
         Illness. St. Louis, Missouri: C.V. Mosby Co.

Index

The numbers in this index refer to entry numbers, not page numbers.

About the Compiler

ERNEST L. ABEL is a Research Scientist V at the Research Institute on Alcoholism in Buffalo, New York. He has prepared several bibliographies on health-related subjects, including *A Comprehensive Guide to the Cannabis Literature* (Greenwood Press, 1979), *Alcohol and Reproduction* (Greenwood Press, 1982), *A Marihuana Dictionary* (Greenwood Press, 1981), *Alcohol and the Elderly* (Greenwood Press, 1980, with Grace M. Barnes), and *Smoking and Reproduction* (Greenwood Press, 1982). His articles have appeared in *Science, Nature,* and *Neurobehavioral Teratology.*